Independent NASM CPT Study Guide 2027-2028:

600 Realistic Practice Questions with Detailed Rationale for Certified Personal Trainer Success

AF879957

Yolanda Mensah

Author Introduction

The Certified Personal Trainer (CPT) examination represents a foundational credential within the health and fitness industry, validating professional competence in exercise science, program design, client assessment, and safe training practices. As personal trainers assume responsibility for guiding individuals toward improved physical performance, injury prevention, and overall wellness, the examination evaluates a candidate's ability to apply evidence-based principles in diverse fitness settings. Mastery of anatomy, physiology, biomechanics, nutrition fundamentals, and risk management is essential to ensure client safety and measurable outcomes.

The author of this study guide brings extensive expertise in exercise physiology, strength and conditioning principles, and professional fitness instruction standards. With a comprehensive understanding of functional assessment protocols, individualized program development, corrective exercise strategies, and client-centered coaching methodologies, the author has structured this material to reflect the full scope of professional personal training practice. Emphasis is placed on integrating scientific principles with applied training scenarios, reinforcing the ability to evaluate movement patterns, design progressive programming, adapt sessions to client needs, and maintain professional and ethical boundaries. The author's disciplined methodology ensures that foundational science is consistently translated into practical application consistent with industry expectations.

Development of this guide followed systematic analysis of official examination content outlines and competency domains. Each section aligns directly with tested areas, including client intake and screening, exercise technique and instruction, program design and modification, nutrition considerations, and professional responsibility. Structured domain mapping and blueprint alignment were employed to ensure fidelity to exam specifications. Practice questions were developed to reflect exam-level rigor, emphasizing critical thinking, applied biomechanics, safety screening, and evidence-based decision-making. Editorial review and quality assurance processes were implemented to ensure technical accuracy, terminological precision, and alignment with recognized health and fitness standards.

This resource reflects the author's commitment to advancing professional excellence within the fitness profession. Designed as a comprehensive and independent preparation tool, it supports candidates in demonstrating the scientific knowledge, applied competence, and ethical responsibility required for success on the Certified Personal Trainer examination and for effective practice in the health and fitness industry.

Table of Contents

Copyright Notice

© 2026. All rights reserved. This publication is protected by United States copyright law and by international treaties and conventions. No portion of this book may be reproduced, distributed, transmitted, stored in a retrieval system, or transmitted in any form or by any means—electronic, mechanical, photocopying, recording, scanning, or otherwise—without prior written permission from the publisher, except as permitted under applicable copyright law. Brief quotations for review, academic citation, or scholarly analysis are permitted provided proper attribution is included.

This publication has been developed as an independent educational resource designed to support preparation for professional certification and licensure examinations. The material is based on structured analysis of publicly available examination outlines, industry standards, and generally accepted professional practices current at the time of publication. While every effort has been made to ensure accuracy, clarity, and completeness, the author and publisher make no representations or warranties regarding errors, omissions, or subsequent changes to examination requirements, regulatory standards, or professional guidelines.

This work is not affiliated with, endorsed by, sponsored by, or approved by any certification board, licensing authority, or examination provider. Any trademarks, service marks, registered trademarks, trade names, or organizational names referenced in this publication are the property of their respective owners and are used solely for identification purposes.

The author and publisher disclaim any liability for loss, injury, claim, or damages arising directly or indirectly from the use or application of the information contained in this book. Readers are responsible for verifying current standards, regulations, and examination requirements through official sources.

Disclaimer

NASM CPT® is a registered trademark of the National Academy of Sports Medicine (NASM). This publication is an independent study tool and is not affiliated with or endorsed by NASM®.

Chapter 1: Basic and Applied Sciences and Nutritional Concepts

The Foundations of Human Structure and Function

Every aspect of movement begins with an understanding of human structure and the organization of life from the cellular to the systemic level. The body is composed of millions of cells working collectively to maintain homeostasis, the dynamic equilibrium that supports life. These cells form tissues, tissues form organs, and organs unite into systems that perform specialized functions such as movement, circulation, or digestion. In the context of personal training, this organization determines how forces are produced, absorbed, and transferred during exercise. Understanding the relationships between structure and function allows trainers to predict how the body responds to mechanical stress, energy demand, and environmental changes. For example, skeletal muscle fibers are designed for contraction, but their efficiency depends on oxygen delivery from the cardiovascular system and the neural signals that initiate motion. The integration of these systems transforms theory into coordinated performance. When viewed through this scientific lens, human movement becomes a symphony of biological cooperation—each system contributing to the rhythm of strength, stability, and adaptation. Recognizing these interconnections forms the bedrock of evidence-based fitness practice.

Chemical and Cellular Basis of Human Life

Beneath the visible mechanics of movement lies a complex network of chemical reactions that sustain energy flow and tissue maintenance. Every contraction of a muscle or firing of a neuron is powered by biochemical transformations at the cellular level. The body's essential elements—carbon, hydrogen, oxygen, and nitrogen—combine in specific ratios to build the molecules of life: proteins, carbohydrates, lipids, and nucleic acids. Within cells, these molecules participate in reactions that generate adenosine triphosphate, or ATP, the currency of energy. Trainers who appreciate these chemical processes can better understand fatigue, recovery, and nutrition-based performance strategies. The cell membrane regulates nutrient exchange, while organelles such as mitochondria serve as energy factories, converting food substrates into usable fuel through aerobic and anaerobic pathways. Cellular respiration, involving glycolysis, the Krebs cycle, and oxidative phosphorylation, illustrates how nutrients are transformed into movement. The cellular environment must also maintain pH balance and electrolyte distribution, both crucial for muscular and neural function. Any disruption to these delicate processes can hinder exercise performance or adaptation. Thus, a solid grasp of basic chemistry and cellular biology provides trainers with insight into the invisible but essential energy systems that sustain every human action.

The Nervous System and Movement Control

The nervous system orchestrates all voluntary and involuntary motion. It interprets environmental information, sends commands to muscles, and refines movement through feedback and adaptation. This control begins with the sensory division, which collects data about position, pressure, and temperature, and extends through the motor division, which directs the muscular response. The central nervous system, composed of the brain and spinal cord, acts as the command center, while the peripheral system transmits signals to and from body structures. Each motor neuron communicates with muscle fibers at neuromuscular junctions, forming motor units whose coordinated firing produces precise motion.

Repetition and practice refine these neural pathways, improving synchronization, balance, and reaction time. Neural adaptation precedes muscular growth, explaining why early strength gains often occur before visible hypertrophy. The nervous system also influences posture and movement efficiency through reflexes and proprioception—internal sensory feedback that informs body awareness. Trainers who understand neural integration can coach correct technique, prevent compensatory movement patterns, and promote stability. Efficient communication between the brain and muscles defines the quality of human movement and underscores why motor learning is as vital as mechanical strength in achieving long-term fitness outcomes.

The Muscular System and Energy Dynamics

Muscles convert stored chemical energy into mechanical force, generating motion, maintaining posture, and stabilizing joints. Each skeletal muscle contains bundles of fibers organized into fascicles surrounded by connective tissue layers that provide strength and elasticity. Within every fiber, myofibrils consist of repeating sarcomeres—the fundamental units of contraction. Actin and myosin filaments slide past one another in a coordinated cycle powered by ATP, a process controlled by calcium release from the sarcoplasmic reticulum. The efficiency of this sliding filament mechanism determines muscular strength and endurance. Muscle fibers vary in their physiological properties: slow-twitch fibers rely on oxidative metabolism and sustain long-duration effort, while fast-twitch fibers generate high force rapidly through anaerobic pathways. Regular training modifies the functional capacity of these fibers, increasing mitochondrial density, capillarization, and enzyme activity. Muscles operate in kinetic chains, working together to produce smooth, controlled movement. The balance between agonists, antagonists, and stabilizers ensures joint integrity and optimal power transfer. Understanding these relationships enables trainers to prescribe exercises that promote balanced development and prevent overuse. Ultimately, the muscular system embodies the physical expression of the body's energy systems, transforming biochemical potential into visible motion and performance.

The Skeletal Framework of Motion

The skeletal system provides the rigid framework upon which all movement is built. It supports body weight, protects internal organs, and serves as an anchor for muscle attachment. Bones are living tissues that continuously remodel in response to mechanical stress, maintaining strength through the coordinated activity of osteoblasts and osteoclasts. This process, known as Wolff's law, explains how consistent resistance training increases bone density and structural resilience. Joints, classified by movement type and connective structure, allow controlled motion across the body's axes. Synovial joints, such as the shoulder or knee, facilitate dynamic movement through lubrication and cartilage cushioning, while fibrous and cartilaginous joints provide stability in less mobile regions. The skeletal and muscular systems operate as a mechanical partnership: bones act as levers, joints as fulcrums, and muscles as force generators. Understanding lever mechanics—such as how resistance and effort arms determine torque—allows precise adjustment of exercise intensity and range of motion. Additionally, the axial skeleton supports posture and protects vital organs, while the appendicular skeleton enables locomotion and interaction with the environment. Trainers who grasp skeletal biomechanics can optimize performance while safeguarding joint health, turning knowledge of structure into a tool for longevity and movement precision.

The Endocrine Regulation of Performance

Beneath the muscular and neural actions of training lies a finely tuned endocrine system that governs adaptation and recovery. Hormones act as chemical messengers, circulating through the bloodstream to regulate metabolism, growth, and tissue repair. During exercise, the hypothalamus and pituitary glands coordinate a cascade of hormonal responses that mobilize energy stores, increase heart rate, and enhance nutrient transport. Cortisol and epinephrine elevate glucose availability for immediate fuel, while growth hormone and testosterone stimulate protein synthesis and muscle remodeling. Insulin and glucagon maintain glucose balance, ensuring continuous energy supply during training and recovery. The endocrine response varies with exercise intensity, duration, and type, illustrating the body's adaptability. Chronic stress or inadequate recovery can disrupt hormonal equilibrium, leading to fatigue or reduced performance. Trainers must recognize the significance of rest, nutrition, and progressive overload in maintaining healthy endocrine balance. Understanding this internal communication network allows more effective programming and recovery strategies, ensuring that clients adapt productively rather than accumulate stress. The endocrine system thus serves as the unseen regulator of performance, translating training stimuli into lasting physiological change through precise hormonal orchestration.

The Cardiorespiratory System in Exercise

The integration of cardiovascular and respiratory function sustains the delivery of oxygen and nutrients to working tissues. The heart, composed of specialized cardiac muscle, operates as a dual pump that maintains continuous circulation. Oxygenated blood travels from the left ventricle through systemic arteries, while deoxygenated blood returns via veins to the right side for pulmonary exchange. The respiratory system complements this cycle by facilitating gas exchange within the alveoli, where oxygen diffuses into capillaries and carbon dioxide is expelled. Exercise challenges these systems to operate at higher efficiency, increasing cardiac output, stroke volume, and respiratory rate. Through endurance training, adaptations occur: the heart muscle strengthens, capillary networks expand, and mitochondrial density increases, all of which enhance oxygen utilization. Proper cardiorespiratory function supports energy production during both aerobic and anaerobic efforts, influencing fatigue thresholds and recovery time. Trainers who understand these mechanisms can prescribe intensity zones that match a client's conditioning level and goals. Efficient oxygen transport underlies stamina, speed, and metabolic resilience, making this system central to all aspects of fitness performance and overall vitality.

Nutritional Concepts and Energy Balance

Nutrition provides the raw materials for movement, recovery, and cellular repair. Understanding how macronutrients and micronutrients support exercise physiology enables trainers to guide clients toward balanced, sustainable habits. Carbohydrates serve as the primary energy source, stored as glycogen in muscles and liver tissue. Fats supply concentrated energy during prolonged, moderate-intensity activity, while proteins contribute to tissue maintenance and enzyme function. Adequate hydration and electrolyte balance are equally essential for neuromuscular coordination and thermoregulation. Caloric balance—matching intake with expenditure—determines weight maintenance, while positive or negative balances lead to gain or loss respectively. Beyond energy, micronutrients such as calcium, iron, and B-vitamins facilitate metabolic reactions and oxygen transport. Trainers do not prescribe specific diets but educate clients on fundamental principles, encouraging whole foods, appropriate portion control, and nutrient timing aligned with activity level. Understanding how food supports the physiological processes of adaptation bridges the gap between nutrition and training. The synergy of diet and exercise determines how effectively the body recovers, grows, and sustains long-term health.

Homeostasis and the Principles of Adaptation

The human body strives to maintain stability through constant internal regulation, a process known as homeostasis. During exercise, temperature, pH, and energy demands shift rapidly, requiring coordinated adjustments across systems. The nervous and endocrine networks detect deviations and trigger corrective responses to restore equilibrium. Over time, these repeated challenges lead to adaptation—the body's improved capacity to handle future stress. Muscular strength, cardiovascular endurance, and metabolic efficiency all result from this adaptive cycle. The principle of progressive overload operates within this biological framework: gradual increases in demand stimulate further adaptation, while excessive stress can lead to overtraining or injury. Recovery periods allow systems to repair and strengthen, reinforcing balance. Trainers who respect this balance craft programs that challenge the body without overwhelming it. Homeostasis is thus not a static condition but a dynamic process that underlies every improvement in fitness. Mastering this concept empowers professionals to design interventions that harness the body's natural capacity for renewal, achieving results grounded in science rather than guesswork.

Integrating Science into Professional Practice

The ultimate goal of understanding applied sciences is to translate knowledge into safe, effective, and individualized training experiences. Professional trainers must connect anatomy, physiology, and nutrition into a unified framework that supports each client's goals and limitations. This integration begins with assessment and continues through program design, monitoring, and adaptation. A scientifically informed trainer evaluates movement patterns, identifies imbalances, and selects interventions that align with the client's physiological readiness. Effective communication ensures clients understand the rationale behind each decision, fostering trust and adherence. The science of movement is not confined to textbooks; it lives in every coaching cue, rest interval, and post-session reflection. By blending theoretical mastery with human empathy, trainers become both educators and motivators. In practice, this integration transforms the gym floor into a classroom of applied science where progress is measured not only in performance but in confidence and health. The professional who embodies this synthesis elevates the field, demonstrating that knowledge and care together form the foundation of true fitness leadership.

Chapter 2: Assessment

The Purpose and Philosophy of Fitness Assessment

Assessment represents the scientific foundation of every client-centered training program. It provides measurable data that define a client's physiological status, functional capacity, and movement quality before any intervention begins. For the fitness professional, assessment is not a single event but a continuous process that evolves with the client's progress. It transforms observation into informed decision-making. The philosophy behind assessment is rooted in the principle of "first, move well—then move often." This means establishing a baseline of functional integrity before applying progressive overload. By collecting both subjective and objective data, trainers gain insight into the client's history, motivation, and potential risk factors. Effective assessment bridges the gap between health screening and program design, allowing for targeted prescriptions that align with a client's needs rather than assumptions. In practice, assessment empowers both trainer and client to work from evidence, track measurable outcomes, and refine the path to improvement. It eliminates guesswork and fosters accountability, creating a professional framework that distinguishes scientific fitness coaching from recreational exercise.

Preparticipation Health Screening and Client Readiness

Before physical assessment begins, trainers must ensure the client is medically and physically ready for exercise. The preparticipation screening process evaluates risk factors related to cardiovascular, metabolic, or orthopedic conditions. Instruments such as the Physical Activity Readiness Questionnaire (PAR-Q) and health history forms are used to identify symptoms or contraindications that may require medical clearance. The screening also includes questions about medications, lifestyle habits, stress levels, and previous injuries. This initial review forms the ethical and legal foundation of practice, ensuring client safety and aligning with NASM's scope of practice. Readiness extends beyond physical condition—it includes psychological readiness and commitment. Understanding motivation and perceived barriers helps trainers tailor coaching strategies to enhance adherence. Through systematic screening, trainers categorize clients into low, moderate, or high risk, guiding whether they may proceed with standard assessments or require referral to a healthcare provider. The goal is prevention: identifying potential complications before they manifest during training. This step embodies professional responsibility, demonstrating that assessment begins with safety, respect for individual differences, and collaboration with the broader healthcare network.

Subjective Assessment: Building the Client Profile

Subjective assessment focuses on gathering personal and historical data that shape the client's fitness narrative. Information on occupation, daily activity, sleep, and nutrition reveals patterns that influence movement and recovery. A sedentary desk worker, for example, may exhibit postural deviations and reduced hip mobility due to prolonged sitting, while a physically active laborer might show repetitive stress patterns from overuse. The subjective phase also includes exploring psychosocial elements—stress perception, goal orientation, and readiness to change. Understanding these factors enables trainers to identify root causes of dysfunction beyond the musculoskeletal system. The subjective assessment also sets the tone for rapport and trust. Through open-ended questions, the trainer demonstrates empathy and professionalism, fostering honesty in responses. By connecting lifestyle insights with future testing outcomes, trainers can better interpret objective data within real-life context. A thorough subjective evaluation transforms numerical scores into meaningful stories about human behavior, revealing not just what a client can do, but why certain limitations exist. This deeper understanding allows for programming that honors both the science of movement and the psychology of motivation.

Objective Assessment: Measuring the Body in Motion

Objective assessment translates the art of observation into quantifiable metrics. This phase evaluates measurable components of fitness such as heart rate, blood pressure, body composition, postural alignment, and movement control. Each parameter offers clues about systemic health and biomechanical efficiency. Resting heart rate and blood pressure provide insight into cardiovascular conditioning and recovery status, while circumference and skinfold measurements reveal patterns of fat distribution and muscle development. Postural assessments expose deviations—rounded shoulders, anterior pelvic tilt, or knee valgus—that may indicate muscular imbalance or kinetic chain dysfunction. Movement assessments, such as squats, pushes, and pulls, reveal compensations and coordination deficits. Objective testing provides the raw data needed to design personalized exercise prescriptions. Consistency and accuracy are paramount; trainers should apply standardized procedures, calibrate equipment, and document results clearly for comparison over time. Objective evaluation transforms assumptions into measurable facts, allowing the professional to identify strengths and weaknesses, prioritize interventions, and demonstrate progress with tangible evidence.

Static Postural Assessment and Alignment Principles

Posture serves as the blueprint for functional movement. Static postural assessment involves observing the client's body alignment in a relaxed standing position from anterior, lateral, and posterior views. Trainers evaluate joint alignment of the head, shoulders, spine, hips, knees, and ankles to detect muscular imbalances or asymmetries. Common deviations—such as forward head posture, excessive lumbar curvature, or pronated feet—reveal patterns of overactive and underactive muscles along the kinetic chain. These deviations are not merely aesthetic; they influence movement efficiency, load distribution, and injury susceptibility. For example, a forward head posture can disrupt scapular mechanics and breathing patterns, while pelvic tilt affects gait and core stability. Through careful observation, trainers interpret these structural patterns and relate them to functional outcomes. Postural assessment is a starting point for corrective exercise strategy. It provides a visual map of how everyday habits—sitting, lifting, or standing—shape long-term alignment. Recognizing these details enables trainers to restore balance, improve mobility, and lay the groundwork for optimal movement execution.

Dynamic and Functional Movement Assessment

Dynamic assessment examines how the body performs under motion, revealing compensatory strategies and neuromuscular control. Using tools such as the overhead squat, single-leg squat, and pushing or pulling assessments, trainers observe the integration of the nervous, muscular, and skeletal systems in real time. Each movement pattern serves as a diagnostic window into stability, mobility, and coordination. A collapsing knee during a squat, for instance, may signal hip abductor weakness or limited ankle dorsiflexion. Unlike static assessment, which identifies structure, dynamic evaluation reveals function. Trainers analyze the quality, timing, and symmetry of movement, not just the end result. The goal is to identify faulty mechanics before they evolve into overuse injuries. Functional assessments also include performance-based tests such as step-ups or balance challenges, depending on the client's level. Mastery of movement quality precedes intensity, reinforcing NASM's principle of building stability before strength. By addressing dysfunction through corrective strategies early, trainers ensure safer progression into advanced training phases. Dynamic assessment thus bridges anatomy with performance, transforming observation into proactive movement correction.

Performance Assessment and Athletic Evaluation

Performance assessment measures the capabilities that define physical fitness—strength, endurance, flexibility, speed, and power. Unlike functional screening, performance testing focuses on quantifying specific capacities relevant to the client's goals. Common tests include push-up or bench press evaluations for muscular endurance, vertical jump and medicine ball toss for power, and timed sprints or agility drills for coordination. These tests are selected according to the client's level, ensuring they complement rather than compromise foundational stability. The NASM approach emphasizes that performance results must always be interpreted within the context of movement quality; strong performance cannot compensate for poor mechanics. Trainers record baseline data to track improvement and identify training adaptations over time. Performance assessment also contributes to motivation by providing measurable benchmarks of success. When integrated into the broader assessment framework, it supports progressive overload by defining appropriate training intensities. In advanced populations such as athletes, these evaluations refine conditioning strategies and minimize injury risk by aligning physical potential with biomechanical integrity.

The Functional Movement Screen in Personal Training

The Functional Movement Screen (FMS) provides a standardized method for evaluating fundamental movement patterns. It measures mobility, stability, and symmetry across seven key exercises, including the deep squat, hurdle step, inline lunge, shoulder mobility reach, active straight-leg raise, trunk stability push-up, and rotary stability test. Each movement is scored on a scale reflecting quality and compensation. The goal is not competition but detection—identifying limitations that may predispose clients to inefficiency or injury. The FMS complements NASM's assessment model by offering a visual and reproducible baseline for movement competency. Trainers use results to prioritize corrective exercise before applying load or intensity. The system's simplicity belies its depth: small deviations often reveal underlying dysfunctions within the kinetic chain. For example, asymmetry in the hurdle step may point to hip mobility deficits or core instability. The FMS transforms assessment into a preventive tool, helping trainers refine exercise selection and monitor improvement. Its application underscores that safe performance begins with quality movement, making it indispensable in professional fitness practice.

Interpreting Data and Communicating Results

Assessment is only valuable when data are interpreted and communicated effectively. The trainer's role extends beyond collecting numbers to translating results into meaningful insights. Patterns of imbalance, asymmetry, or deficiency must be explained in language clients understand, emphasizing empowerment rather than judgment. Visual aids such as progress charts or movement diagrams can help illustrate improvement over time. Clear communication strengthens trust and motivates adherence. When discussing results, trainers should connect findings directly to the client's goals—how improved mobility supports running efficiency or how posture correction reduces discomfort. Interpretation also involves identifying priorities; not every deficit requires immediate intervention. By ranking issues according to impact on safety and performance, trainers can implement phased strategies. Effective interpretation turns assessment into education, encouraging clients to take ownership of their progress. The professional's ability to translate science into simple, actionable feedback distinguishes expert coaching from mechanical instruction, ensuring assessment remains a dynamic and motivating experience.

Integrating Assessment into Continuous Program Design

Assessment is not a one-time event but an ongoing dialogue between the body and its response to training. Each phase of the OPT model—stabilization, strength, and power—requires re-evaluation to measure adaptation and prevent plateau. Trainers must revisit both subjective and objective data to confirm that progress aligns with intended outcomes. Changes in performance, posture, or wellness indicators often reveal whether programming variables are appropriate or need adjustment. Continuous assessment also supports long-term client retention by demonstrating accountability and professional rigor. Documented improvements in strength, endurance, or movement quality validate the effectiveness of coaching and reinforce motivation. Importantly, reassessment ensures that the program evolves with the client's capacity rather than remaining static. By embedding assessment as a recurring practice, trainers uphold the principle of scientific training: observe, apply, evaluate, and refine. The result is a system that honors individuality, ensures safety, and transforms exercise into a process of lifelong learning and measurable growth.

Download Audio File and Flashcards

Chapter 3: Exercise Technique and Training Instruction

The Principles of Safe and Effective Movement

Proper exercise technique is the cornerstone of all training programs, ensuring that every repetition reinforces safe, efficient, and purposeful movement. The trainer's role is to blend biomechanical precision with client awareness, guiding posture, range of motion, and alignment through every phase of the exercise. Each repetition becomes both a diagnostic and corrective opportunity. Poor mechanics not only reduce training efficiency but also accumulate stress that may lead to injury. Therefore, instruction must begin with fundamental movement principles: neutral spine alignment, controlled joint motion, and the stabilization of the core before limb movement. Mastery of these fundamentals enhances motor control and allows progressive loading without compromising form. Trainers must also adapt technique to client anatomy and ability, adjusting stance, grip, or leverage as needed. Correct technique is more than memorizing form—it represents mindful movement executed with intent. Through consistent instruction, the trainer transforms exercise from random effort into structured skill development, establishing the technical foundation upon which performance and safety depend.

The Kinetic Chain and Integrated Movement

Human movement occurs through a coordinated interaction between the muscular, skeletal, and nervous systems—collectively known as the kinetic chain. Every exercise, whether a squat, press, or pull, requires multiple systems working in harmony to transfer force efficiently. When one link of the chain is weak or overactive, compensations appear that alter movement quality. Trainers must therefore view each exercise not in isolation but as part of a connected system. For example, tight hip flexors may cause excessive lumbar arching during squats, while underactive gluteal muscles can limit power generation and joint alignment. The principle of integrated movement emphasizes that stabilization and mobility are interdependent qualities: stability allows mobility, and mobility supports stability. Instruction must guide clients toward balanced activation patterns that respect this dynamic. Observing movement through the lens of the kinetic chain helps trainers identify inefficiencies early and teach corrective mechanics. Ultimately, training the chain as a unit enhances coordination, minimizes injury risk, and builds the functional strength that transfers seamlessly to everyday activity.

Foundations of Integrated Flexibility and Mobility

Flexibility and mobility training serve as prerequisites for effective resistance and power performance. A client who lacks adequate range of motion cannot achieve proper technique, regardless of strength or intent. Flexibility refers to the extensibility of soft tissue, while mobility reflects the ability of joints to move freely through intended planes. Both are influenced by neuromuscular control, connective tissue elasticity, and habitual posture. Techniques such as self-myofascial release, static stretching, and dynamic mobility drills help restore balance between overactive and underactive muscles. Trainers should teach flexibility within the context of movement preparation, not as isolated stretching routines. A dynamic warm-up, incorporating controlled, sport-specific motions, activates the nervous system while improving joint readiness. Flexibility instruction must respect individual variation; forcing range through passive means may disrupt joint integrity. Effective mobility work supports symmetrical movement, improves circulation, and reduces compensatory stress. When integrated into every session, flexibility instruction prepares the body for technical precision, reinforcing the idea that mobility is not optional but essential to movement mastery.

Cueing Strategies for Effective Instruction

The art of cueing transforms technical knowledge into client understanding. An effective cue bridges the gap between biomechanics and action, guiding movement through concise, purposeful communication. Trainers employ three primary cueing styles: visual, auditory, and kinesthetic. Visual cues demonstrate ideal posture or range; auditory cues use rhythm, imagery, or verbal emphasis; kinesthetic cues involve tactile guidance when appropriate. The best instructors tailor their cueing language to each learner's sensory preference and comprehension level. Overloading clients with excessive instruction can cause confusion, so cues should be clear, sequential, and outcome-oriented. For instance, instead of "keep your knees from caving in," a trainer might say, "press the floor apart with your feet." This positive framing directs action rather than correction. As clients advance, external cues—focusing on movement outcomes like "drive the ground away"—promote automatic control and performance efficiency. Effective cueing requires presence and observation, ensuring each message resonates with timing and purpose. Through consistent and precise cues, trainers cultivate body awareness and empower clients to internalize proper movement patterns.

Resistance Training Technique and Execution

Resistance training demands an exact balance between control and intensity. Each exercise must be performed with deliberate rhythm, proper alignment, and complete range of motion suited to the individual's flexibility and stability. The trainer's instruction focuses on start and finish positions, grip variations, breathing rhythm, and tempo control. During concentric motion, the client generates force smoothly, avoiding momentum or abrupt acceleration. The eccentric phase, where muscles lengthen under tension, should be controlled to enhance strength and joint stability. Trainers must reinforce that effective lifting is about mastery, not maximal load. Teaching clients to "own" every inch of movement ensures consistent neuromuscular recruitment and minimizes energy leaks. Proper spotting and setup are critical, especially in multi-joint lifts like bench presses or squats. Each repetition represents an opportunity to reinforce correct motor sequencing. By combining biomechanical understanding with attentive coaching, trainers ensure every resistance exercise becomes a tool for safe, progressive adaptation rather than mechanical repetition.

Core Stabilization and Movement Efficiency

The concept of core training extends beyond abdominal strengthening; it represents the integration of deep stabilizing muscles that maintain posture and transfer force. The core includes the lumbar spine, pelvis, and hip complex—collectively forming the foundation for all limb motion. When the core is stable, energy transfers efficiently from the lower to the upper body, preventing compensatory strain. Instruction in core stability emphasizes alignment, controlled breathing, and sequential activation. Exercises such as planks, bridges, and controlled rotational drills enhance proprioception and coordination across multiple planes. Trainers should teach clients to stabilize before mobilizing, ensuring that dynamic movement emerges from a solid base. Core instruction progresses from static control to dynamic challenges, always prioritizing form over volume. A strong core not only improves strength expression but also protects the spine during heavy resistance training. By integrating core training into every session, trainers build resilience that supports optimal performance across all exercise modalities.

Teaching Proper Breathing and Intra-Abdominal Control

Breathing is often overlooked but profoundly influences performance, posture, and safety. During resistance exercise, proper breathing stabilizes the torso and prevents excessive internal pressure that could strain the cardiovascular system. Trainers teach clients to inhale during the eccentric phase and exhale during the concentric, promoting rhythm and oxygen delivery. In heavy lifts, advanced clients may use the Valsalva maneuver—a brief breath hold—to increase intra-abdominal pressure and spinal rigidity, but only under controlled supervision. Poor breathing patterns, such as shallow chest respiration, limit core engagement and fatigue the accessory muscles of respiration. Diaphragmatic breathing enhances oxygen efficiency and reinforces trunk control, especially during compound movements. Instruction must integrate breath awareness into every repetition, helping clients maintain composure under load. By synchronizing respiration with effort, trainers foster endurance, reduce dizziness or strain, and promote mindful exercise execution. Correct breathing transforms lifting into a coordinated act of stability and flow rather than brute exertion.

Teaching Balance, Stability, and Control

Balance training develops the body's ability to maintain equilibrium during movement and under external load. It relies on sensory feedback from the visual, vestibular, and proprioceptive systems. Trainers teach balance progressively, beginning with stable surfaces and advancing toward dynamic or unstable environments. Controlled instability—such as using balance boards or single-leg stances—challenges coordination and enhances joint stabilization. However, instability must never replace sound biomechanics; it is a tool to refine, not complicate, technique. Balance instruction integrates postural alignment, controlled tempo, and breathing awareness to reinforce motor control. The ability to stabilize the body under shifting demands directly influences strength development and athletic performance. Each balance exercise becomes a test of control rather than risk. When mastered, balance training enhances confidence, proprioception, and muscular coordination, supporting every other aspect of the fitness continuum. In professional practice, teaching balance ensures that strength expresses itself as usable, functional stability across all planes of movement.

Movement Tempo and Training Variables

Tempo governs how muscles produce and control force across the eccentric, isometric, and concentric phases of an exercise. Trainers use tempo notation to describe time under tension—for example, 3/1/2 represents a three-second lowering phase, a one-second pause, and a two-second lift. Controlling tempo enhances muscle activation, reinforces stability, and modulates intensity without changing external load. Slower tempos increase time under tension and improve control, while faster tempos develop power and neuromuscular responsiveness. Instruction in tempo teaches clients awareness of pacing and quality of motion. It also connects with broader training variables such as volume, rest intervals, and intensity within the OPT model. A consistent tempo allows trainers to evaluate fatigue and technical endurance objectively. Educating clients on tempo cultivates discipline and precision, reminding them that mastery in movement arises from rhythm as much as from resistance. Through intentional pacing, the trainer shapes performance into a deliberate, efficient, and safe physical expression.

Professional Instruction and Coaching Presence

Technical knowledge alone does not create effective instruction; the trainer's presence transforms information into experience. Professional instruction involves observation, empathy, and real-time adjustment. Trainers must read subtle cues—facial tension, posture shifts, or breathing irregularities—to determine when to correct or encourage. Coaching presence is built on calm authority and communication clarity, ensuring clients feel supported yet challenged. Effective instruction maintains consistency without rigidity, adapting technique cues to each client's learning style and feedback response. The trainer's demeanor reinforces confidence and safety, which directly influences performance outcomes. Each session becomes a conversation between science and intuition, where the trainer applies analytical reasoning within a human context. Professional instruction also means maintaining ethical boundaries, providing corrections through verbal or visual demonstration before physical contact. Ultimately, great coaching merges knowledge, timing, and empathy—turning the exercise floor into a place where learning, motivation, and precision coexist in seamless harmony.

Chapter 4: Program Design

The Science and Philosophy of Program Design

Program design is both an art and a science—the strategic process of organizing acute variables and training components to achieve specific client outcomes. Every effective program must rest upon scientific principles of adaptation while remaining flexible enough to accommodate individual differences. The trainer's goal is to bridge physiology and practicality, translating theory into structured action. A well-constructed program begins with assessment results and client goals, progresses through evidence-based planning, and concludes with evaluation and refinement. The NASM Optimum Performance Training (OPT) model provides the overarching structure for this process, guiding progression from stabilization to strength and power. Each phase emphasizes specific physiological adaptations—such as endurance, hypertrophy, or maximal force production—while maintaining movement quality. Program design also integrates recovery, nutrition, and psychological readiness, acknowledging that the human body adapts holistically. Ultimately, program design is a dialogue between stimulus and response, where the trainer manipulates volume, intensity, frequency, and rest to elicit desired changes. When applied with precision and creativity, design transforms training from routine exercise into purposeful progression.

Acute Variables and Their Application

Acute variables are the fundamental building blocks of exercise prescription—those adjustable components that define every training session. They include repetitions, sets, intensity, tempo, rest intervals, volume, and frequency. Manipulating these factors determines the physiological adaptation targeted, whether endurance, hypertrophy, strength, or power. For instance, lower intensities with higher repetitions emphasize muscular endurance, while high-load, low-repetition schemes stimulate neural and hypertrophic adaptations. The interplay among variables must always reflect the client's capacity, goals, and recovery ability. Trainers apply these variables systematically within the OPT model's phase structure, using stabilization-focused training to build movement integrity before progressing to heavier loads. The correct manipulation of tempo and rest is particularly vital; shorter rests maintain metabolic stress, whereas longer intervals allow neural recovery for maximal efforts. Acute variables interact like instruments in an orchestra—each must be tuned precisely to achieve harmony in adaptation. Mastery of these elements enables trainers to craft sessions that are efficient, measurable, and safe, ensuring consistent progress and reduced risk of overtraining.

Understanding the OPT Model and Phase Progression

The Optimum Performance Training (OPT) model serves as NASM's systematic framework for integrated training. It is structured into three progressive levels—stabilization, strength, and power—each containing distinct phases with specific goals. The stabilization level develops movement efficiency, core control, and postural alignment through controlled, low-load exercises emphasizing form. The strength level expands muscular capacity and introduces overload through the phases of strength endurance, hypertrophy, and maximal strength. Finally, the power level integrates force and velocity, training the body to express strength dynamically. Each level builds upon the previous one, ensuring adaptation without regression. Trainers must guide clients through these stages based on readiness, not arbitrary timelines. Progression is data-driven, determined by mastery of movement and recovery capability. The OPT model exemplifies periodization—the deliberate variation of training stimuli to avoid plateau. Its structured yet adaptable design allows trainers to address diverse goals, from general fitness to elite performance. Through this model, program design becomes an evidence-based pathway rather than a collection of exercises.

Stabilization Endurance Training: The Foundation Phase

Stabilization endurance training represents the first level of physical preparation in the OPT model. Its primary objective is to develop neuromuscular efficiency—the ability of the nervous and muscular systems to work synergistically to maintain balance and posture during movement. Exercises emphasize controlled tempo, minimal external load, and proper alignment under unstable conditions. This phase enhances joint stability, muscular coordination, and core strength, laying the groundwork for safe progression. Common modalities include balance work, bodyweight resistance, suspension training, and light free-weight exercises performed in circuits with limited rest. By improving endurance of stabilizing musculature, the body gains the ability to maintain alignment under fatigue. Clients in this phase learn how to move efficiently rather than simply exert effort. Trainers should prioritize movement quality over quantity, ensuring the client can stabilize before generating force. This foundation phase instills discipline in form, cultivates awareness, and prevents future imbalances. Stabilization endurance is not a beginner's phase—it is the universal starting point for every athlete and client seeking longevity and performance.

Strength Development and Hypertrophy Programming

The strength level of training focuses on enhancing force production, muscle volume, and joint integrity through progressively heavier loads. Within this stage, hypertrophy and maximal strength subphases target different but complementary outcomes. Hypertrophy programming manipulates volume and intensity to stimulate muscular growth through mechanical tension and metabolic stress. Moderate-to-high loads, controlled tempos, and reduced rest intervals encourage cellular adaptation and fiber enlargement. The maximal strength phase advances load further to train the nervous system's ability to recruit motor units efficiently. Compound lifts such as squats, deadlifts, and presses form the structural core of these programs. Trainers apply the principle of progressive overload—gradually increasing resistance or total volume to challenge adaptation safely. Strength development requires balance between intensity and recovery; insufficient rest can limit progress, while excessive volume risks overtraining. By integrating strength systematically, the program bridges stability and power, enhancing both muscular architecture and functional performance. Strength is not an isolated quality but the platform upon which every other physical capability depends.

Power and Explosive Performance Training

Power training integrates strength and speed to enhance the body's ability to produce force rapidly. It marks the peak of the OPT model's progression, where previously developed stability and strength converge into dynamic performance. Exercises emphasize explosive intent rather than maximal load, often combining heavy resistance moves with high-velocity actions such as plyometrics or medicine ball throws. The neuromuscular system learns to activate quickly, improving rate of force development and reactive ability. This phase demands technical precision and adequate recovery between bouts, as fatigue compromises coordination. Trainers structure sessions using contrast pairings—such as a heavy squat followed by a jump—to exploit post-activation potentiation and reinforce neural efficiency. Power training also enhances daily functional abilities, improving balance, agility, and quickness. Instruction must focus on control, not recklessness; power is a refined expression of strength under speed, not random explosiveness. When properly programmed, this phase refines the athlete's movement economy and ensures the culmination of adaptive potential developed through earlier stages.

Applying Functional Training and Movement Specificity

Functional training emphasizes movement patterns over isolated muscle actions. Its purpose is to enhance the body's ability to perform real-life tasks efficiently and safely. Trainers design programs around multi-joint, multiplanar movements that mimic natural human motion, such as pushing, pulling, squatting, rotating, and stabilizing. Each exercise integrates balance, coordination, and core control, promoting kinetic chain synergy. Functional training also respects the principle of specificity—adaptations reflect the demands placed on the system. A runner's program differs from that of a weightlifter because each must prepare for unique mechanical and metabolic challenges. Trainers must tailor exercises to reflect the client's occupation, sport, or lifestyle while maintaining foundational movement principles. Stability and posture remain central to execution, ensuring functionality does not devolve into instability. By blending purposeful motion with scientific structure, functional training connects the gym environment to real-world movement. It transforms fitness into capability, ensuring that strength and endurance manifest as practical, usable performance.

Integrating Cardiovascular and Resistance Training

Optimal fitness programming integrates cardiovascular conditioning with resistance training to create balanced physiological adaptation. Cardiovascular exercise enhances oxygen transport, endurance, and metabolic efficiency, while resistance training improves strength, stability, and musculoskeletal resilience. Trainers must coordinate these components strategically, managing fatigue and recovery. For general clients, alternating cardio and resistance days supports both systems without interference. In advanced programming, concurrent training principles—sequencing endurance and strength within the same cycle—demand careful variable management. High-intensity interval training (HIIT) offers time-efficient conditioning and supports fat metabolism, provided recovery and technique are monitored. Heart rate zones guide intensity, ensuring clients remain within appropriate energy system targets. By combining modalities, trainers cultivate comprehensive health and performance: a strong heart supporting strong muscles. Integration also promotes adherence, offering variety and balance. The synergy between cardiovascular and resistance elements underscores the holistic philosophy of program design—training the body as one integrated organism rather than as isolated parts.

Periodization and Adaptation Management

Periodization is the structured manipulation of training variables over time to maximize adaptation and prevent plateau. It divides training into cycles—macro, meso, and micro—each with specific objectives and intensity patterns. Linear periodization progresses from high volume, low intensity to lower volume, higher intensity, while undulating models vary these elements more frequently. The purpose is to balance overload with recovery, avoiding stagnation or overtraining. Trainers monitor physiological and psychological responses to adjust volume or rest as needed. Properly periodized programs enhance motivation by providing measurable milestones and variety. Adaptation management also includes planned deload weeks, during which training volume decreases to allow supercompensation. Whether training recreational clients or athletes, periodization ensures long-term progress and sustainability. It reflects the biological reality that improvement requires fluctuation between stress and restoration. Through intelligent scheduling, trainers transform the abstract science of adaptation into a practical timeline of success and safety.

Individualization and Goal-Oriented Design

Every program must reflect the individuality of the client—their physiology, preferences, experience, and limitations. The trainer's role is to blend scientific principles with personalized strategies. Assessments guide goal setting, which in turn shapes exercise selection, intensity, and progression. A weight-loss client may require higher energy expenditure and endurance work, while an athlete demands power and agility refinement. Individualization also considers lifestyle factors such as sleep, stress, and nutrition, which influence recovery and adaptation. Effective programs maintain flexibility, adjusting to feedback and progress. Trainers must recognize that human performance does not follow a perfect linear path; adaptation occurs through variation and persistence. Goal-oriented design keeps motivation tangible and progress measurable, ensuring that every exercise has purpose. When individuality and science align, training becomes not just effective but meaningful—a personal journey built upon professional structure and trust.

Chapter 5: Considerations in Nutrition

The Role of Nutrition in Human Performance

Nutrition forms the biological foundation upon which every aspect of training and recovery depends. Food provides not only the energy to perform exercise but also the molecular materials required to repair, grow, and adapt. The quality and balance of nutrients consumed determine how effectively the body sustains performance, recovers from fatigue, and maintains long-term health. In fitness coaching, the goal is not to prescribe diets but to educate clients on principles that support their objectives—whether weight management, muscle development, or enhanced endurance. Nutritional science reveals how carbohydrates fuel intense effort, fats sustain prolonged activity, and proteins rebuild tissue after exertion. Hydration maintains cellular function and thermoregulation, while vitamins and minerals orchestrate countless biochemical reactions. Trainers must recognize that inadequate or unbalanced nutrition can impair progress, leading to fatigue, slowed adaptation, and compromised immunity. Effective nutrition instruction aligns with individual needs and training demands, reinforcing that exercise and diet are complementary forces. The combination of physical stimulus and proper fueling transforms effort into lasting performance adaptation.

Energy Balance and Metabolism

Energy balance refers to the relationship between calories consumed and calories expended. This equilibrium dictates whether the body maintains, gains, or loses weight over time. Metabolism encompasses the complex biochemical processes that convert food into usable energy, primarily in the form of adenosine triphosphate (ATP). Basal metabolic rate (BMR) accounts for the majority of energy expenditure, representing the energy required to sustain vital physiological functions at rest. Additional energy is used for digestion—known as the thermic effect of food—and for physical activity, which varies according to intensity and duration. Understanding energy balance allows trainers to guide clients in aligning caloric intake with specific goals. Positive balance supports muscle gain and recovery, while negative balance promotes fat reduction when managed responsibly. The macronutrient composition of the diet influences how efficiently energy is produced and utilized. By teaching clients how metabolism adapts to activity, trainers empower them to make informed choices that sustain energy throughout the day and optimize training outcomes.

Carbohydrates: The Body's Preferred Fuel

Carbohydrates provide the most efficient source of energy for muscular work, particularly during moderate to high-intensity exercise. They are stored as glycogen in muscles and liver tissue and can be rapidly broken down into glucose to fuel ATP production. Adequate carbohydrate intake preserves glycogen stores, delays fatigue, and supports consistent performance. The body's limited glycogen capacity—roughly 300 to 600 grams depending on muscle mass—requires regular replenishment through diet. Complex carbohydrates such as whole grains, fruits, and vegetables provide steady glucose release along with essential fiber and micronutrients. Timing also plays a crucial role: consuming carbohydrates before exercise enhances energy availability, while intake after activity accelerates glycogen resynthesis. Low-carbohydrate diets may impair performance if implemented without consideration for intensity and recovery needs. Trainers must communicate the importance of carbohydrates not as a dietary villain but as the body's primary energy source. When consumed strategically, carbohydrates sustain endurance, sharpen concentration, and ensure efficient metabolic recovery following exercise.

Proteins and the Process of Repair and Adaptation

Protein serves as the structural material for nearly every tissue in the body, making it indispensable for recovery and growth. Composed of amino acids, proteins support muscle repair following resistance training and contribute to enzyme and hormone synthesis. During exercise, especially under caloric deficit or intense workloads, small amounts of protein may also serve as an energy substrate. Daily intake recommendations vary with training type and body composition goals, but general fitness populations benefit from approximately 1.2 to 2.0 grams of protein per kilogram of body weight per day. Sources should include a variety of complete and complementary proteins derived from both animal and plant foods. The timing of intake enhances adaptation: consuming protein within one to two hours post-exercise supports muscle protein synthesis and recovery. Quality matters as much as quantity—proteins rich in leucine and essential amino acids optimize anabolic signaling. Proper protein education helps clients understand that consistent, balanced intake—not excess—is key to muscular health, recovery, and overall metabolic function.

Fats: Energy Reserve and Hormonal Balance

Fats provide the body with a dense and long-lasting energy supply, yielding more than twice the caloric value of carbohydrates or proteins per gram. They play essential roles in hormone production, cell membrane integrity, and nutrient absorption, particularly for fat-soluble vitamins A, D, E, and K. While once misunderstood, dietary fats are now recognized as crucial components of a balanced diet. The emphasis lies in selecting the right types: unsaturated fats from sources such as nuts, seeds, fish, and plant oils support cardiovascular health, while excessive saturated or trans fats can elevate disease risk. During low- to moderate-intensity exercise, fats become the dominant energy substrate, preserving glycogen stores for higher-intensity efforts. Adequate intake ensures hormonal stability, particularly for testosterone and estrogen regulation, which directly influence recovery and adaptation. Educating clients on portion awareness and food sources encourages balanced fat consumption without fear or restriction. The key is moderation and diversity, ensuring that fat intake supports both energy metabolism and long-term wellness.

Micronutrients and the Hidden Foundations of Performance

Micronutrients—vitamins and minerals—operate as catalysts for countless metabolic reactions that sustain life and performance. Although they do not provide energy directly, their presence determines how efficiently macronutrients are processed and utilized. For example, B-vitamins facilitate energy metabolism, calcium and vitamin D maintain bone integrity, and iron enables oxygen transport through hemoglobin. Even mild deficiencies can impair endurance, focus, and recovery. Athletes and active individuals often have elevated micronutrient needs due to increased turnover and sweat loss. Balanced diets rich in fruits, vegetables, lean proteins, and whole grains generally meet these requirements, though some populations may benefit from professional evaluation for supplementation. Trainers should emphasize food-first approaches and refer clients to qualified dietitians for advanced nutritional counseling. Understanding micronutrients helps fitness professionals appreciate the delicate biochemical balance that underpins performance—reminding both trainer and client that peak physical output depends as much on invisible nutrients as on visible effort.

Hydration and Fluid Balance in Exercise

Water is the medium of all physiological function, regulating temperature, nutrient transport, and joint lubrication. Even slight dehydration—equivalent to a one to two percent loss of body weight—can impair performance, cognitive function, and cardiovascular efficiency. Fluid needs vary based on body size, climate, and exercise intensity, but general guidelines suggest drinking steadily throughout the day and replacing fluids lost during activity. Electrolytes such as sodium, potassium, and chloride maintain fluid balance and nerve conduction, making their replenishment critical during prolonged sweating. Trainers should teach clients to monitor hydration status through urine color and thirst cues. Pre-hydrating before exercise and consuming fluids at regular intervals during training help sustain plasma volume and prevent heat-related distress. Water remains the optimal fluid for most conditions, while electrolyte beverages are useful for extended or high-intensity sessions. Hydration education fosters awareness that performance begins at the cellular level, where adequate fluid supports every contraction, heartbeat, and breath.

Ergogenic Aids and Supplementation Awareness

Ergogenic aids encompass substances or techniques that may enhance performance, from caffeine and creatine to specialized recovery methods. While some supplements have strong evidence supporting their efficacy, many are marketed with limited or misleading data. Trainers must adopt a neutral, evidence-informed stance, helping clients evaluate potential benefits and risks while remaining within scope of practice. Creatine monohydrate, for example, consistently demonstrates improvements in short-duration, high-intensity performance, while caffeine enhances endurance and focus. However, misuse or overreliance on supplements can displace attention from nutrition fundamentals. Trainers should advise clients to prioritize whole food nutrition and consult registered dietitians or physicians before supplement use. Awareness of labeling, purity testing, and regulatory standards helps reduce exposure to banned or contaminated substances. Education, not prescription, defines the trainer's role—empowering clients to make safe, informed choices that complement, rather than replace, balanced nutrition and consistent training.

Weight Management and Body Composition Strategies

Effective weight management depends on balancing caloric intake with expenditure while maintaining lean body mass. Trainers should emphasize gradual, sustainable changes rather than extreme restriction or rapid loss. Energy deficits of 300–500 calories per day typically support healthy fat reduction without compromising muscle tissue. Resistance training plays a crucial role in preserving lean mass, while cardiovascular exercise contributes to caloric expenditure and metabolic health. Adequate protein intake and nutrient-dense foods prevent nutrient deficiencies common in restrictive diets. For clients seeking weight gain, caloric surpluses combined with progressive overload and sufficient recovery support muscle hypertrophy. Monitoring progress through body composition rather than scale weight provides a clearer picture of true physiological change. Trainers must also recognize the emotional aspects of weight management, fostering positive body image and self-efficacy. By teaching moderation, patience, and consistency, professionals help clients build sustainable habits that align with both physical health and psychological well-being.

Integrating Nutrition into Training Practice

The effective integration of nutrition education into fitness programming enhances results and accountability. Trainers operate within defined professional boundaries, focusing on general guidelines rather than individualized meal plans. Collaboration with registered dietitians ensures clients receive comprehensive support when specific dietary interventions are needed. Within these boundaries, trainers reinforce key habits: balanced meals, regular hydration, and nutrient timing that supports exercise performance. By aligning nutritional awareness with program phases—fueling stabilization, strength, or power training appropriately—clients experience measurable improvements in energy, endurance, and recovery. Nutrition instruction should remain positive and practical, emphasizing flexibility over perfection. The ultimate objective is empowerment: helping clients understand how daily food choices shape training outcomes. When nutrition and exercise operate in harmony, the result is not only improved physical performance but also enhanced vitality, longevity, and overall quality of life.

Chapter 6: Client Relations and Behavioral Coaching

The Human Connection in Fitness Coaching

At the core of effective training lies a genuine human relationship. The interaction between client and trainer extends far beyond technical instruction; it is a process of trust, empathy, and shared purpose. Every client brings a unique story—shaped by experiences, expectations, and barriers—that must be understood before change can occur. The ability to connect authentically transforms the training environment into a space of safety and growth. Listening without judgment, showing consistency, and respecting autonomy establish the foundation for long-term adherence. Research within behavioral psychology confirms that relational quality predicts success more strongly than program content alone. Clients are more likely to sustain physical activity when they feel understood and supported. The professional trainer therefore acts as both educator and collaborator, fostering confidence through encouragement rather than authority. A strong relational bond turns exercise sessions into meaningful exchanges that reinforce the client's self-efficacy and resilience, ultimately guiding behavior change from external motivation to internal commitment.

Foundations of Behavioral Change Theory

Behavioral change theories explain why individuals adopt, sustain, or abandon exercise habits. Understanding these frameworks enables trainers to tailor interventions that align with each client's readiness and mindset. The **Transtheoretical Model** describes progression through stages—from precontemplation to maintenance—highlighting the dynamic nature of change. The **Self-Determination Theory** emphasizes the fulfillment of three basic psychological needs: autonomy, competence, and relatedness. When these needs are met, motivation shifts from extrinsic rewards to intrinsic satisfaction. **Social Cognitive Theory** further contributes by identifying self-efficacy as the central driver of behavioral persistence. These theories converge on one truth: behavior change is not a linear event but an adaptive process. Trainers who integrate these models into practice recognize that setbacks are part of learning, not failure. Effective coaching involves meeting clients where they are, respecting their pace, and using reinforcement strategies that empower them to take ownership of their goals. By combining empathy with theoretical insight, trainers transform exercise instruction into a structured process of behavioral evolution.

Building Trust and Professional Rapport

Trust is the currency of coaching, earned through reliability, respect, and competence. In the early sessions, clients evaluate not only the trainer's knowledge but also their authenticity and consistency. Rapport develops through small but significant actions—remembering personal details, maintaining punctuality, and honoring confidentiality. A transparent, honest communication style reassures clients that their well-being is the trainer's priority. Demonstrating empathy without pity helps clients feel understood while maintaining professional boundaries. Establishing rapport also means adapting one's demeanor to match the client's comfort level—assertive with confident individuals, patient with anxious beginners. Nonverbal behavior, such as eye contact and posture, reinforces sincerity. When rapport is strong, clients communicate openly about challenges, allowing the trainer to design more effective solutions. Trust transforms coaching from instruction into partnership. It shifts motivation from compliance to collaboration, fostering an environment where clients are willing to take risks, confront limitations, and sustain behavior change with confidence.

Effective Communication and Active Listening

Communication is the mechanism through which knowledge becomes transformation. Active listening is its most vital component—the ability to hear beyond words, capturing emotion and intent. Trainers who listen attentively create psychological safety, signaling that the client's experience matters. Techniques such as reflective statements, open-ended questions, and affirmations demonstrate presence and empathy. For example, responding with "It sounds like you feel frustrated when progress slows" validates emotion while keeping dialogue open. Clear, concise feedback prevents confusion and builds trust. Equally important is matching communication style to the client's preferences: some need detailed explanation, while others thrive on concise direction. Trainers should avoid jargon, maintain positive tone, and invite feedback to ensure mutual understanding. Active listening turns sessions into collaborative discussions rather than lectures. It also reveals hidden motivators or obstacles, enabling more accurate coaching strategies. When communication flows effectively, the client feels valued, understood, and capable—critical conditions for sustainable behavioral change.

Motivational Interviewing: Guiding, Not Telling

Motivational Interviewing (MI) is a counseling approach grounded in empathy and self-determination. Rather than persuading clients to change, MI helps them articulate their own reasons for doing so. The process involves four key skills: **asking open questions**, **affirming strengths**, **reflecting statements**, and **summarizing insights**—known collectively as the OARS framework. This method shifts the trainer's role from instructor to facilitator, encouraging clients to explore ambivalence and strengthen intrinsic motivation. Central to MI is the principle that change is most enduring when it originates from the client's own values. Trainers guide conversation through evoking "change talk," statements that express desire or commitment toward a healthier lifestyle. Resistance is met not with confrontation but with curiosity and empathy. Over time, MI fosters self-efficacy, as clients recognize their agency in decision-making. Applying motivational interviewing within fitness sessions nurtures autonomy and engagement, creating an empowering atmosphere that supports sustainable transformation both inside and outside the gym.

Understanding Motivation and Adherence

Motivation is not static; it fluctuates with context, emotion, and perceived success. Trainers must understand the difference between extrinsic motivators—such as appearance or competition—and intrinsic motivators like enjoyment, mastery, and personal growth. Sustainable exercise adherence depends on shifting the motivational focus inward. Behavioral science shows that autonomy-supportive coaching, where clients feel ownership over choices, increases consistency and satisfaction. Trainers can enhance motivation by setting achievable short-term goals and celebrating incremental success. Positive reinforcement, such as acknowledging effort and progress, strengthens self-efficacy and commitment. Conversely, judgment or unrealistic expectations can erode trust and discourage participation. Understanding motivation means recognizing when a client needs challenge versus when they need reassurance. The skilled coach reads emotional cues and adjusts accordingly. Over time, motivation evolves from external accountability to internal desire, transforming exercise from obligation to self-expression—a transition that marks true behavioral sustainability.

Goal Setting and Self-Monitoring Strategies

Goal setting provides direction, while self-monitoring ensures accountability. Effective goals follow the **SMART** framework—specific, measurable, achievable, relevant, and time-bound. However, beyond structure, goals must resonate emotionally to sustain effort. Trainers assist clients in articulating goals that connect to personal meaning rather than abstract metrics. For instance, "I want to play actively with my children" fosters deeper motivation than "I want to lose ten pounds." Self-monitoring tools—training logs, mobile apps, or progress photos—offer tangible feedback that reinforces accomplishment. Tracking progress builds awareness of patterns and reinforces the link between behavior and outcome. When clients witness measurable improvement, confidence and persistence grow. The trainer's role is to balance challenge with achievability, ensuring that goals remain realistic yet inspiring. Regular review sessions allow recalibration, transforming goals from static targets into evolving milestones. When combined, goal setting and self-monitoring form the behavioral backbone of lasting lifestyle change.

Managing Behavioral Barriers and Relapse Prevention

Behavioral change rarely follows a straight line. Setbacks and lapses are natural components of the adaptation process. Trainers must normalize these experiences and teach clients how to recover without shame or discouragement. Common barriers include time constraints, stress, and self-doubt. Identifying these obstacles early allows for proactive problem-solving. Techniques such as implementation intentions—specific "if-then" plans—help clients anticipate challenges ("If I can't train at the gym, I'll complete a home circuit"). Relapse prevention strategies emphasize flexibility rather than perfection. When a setback occurs, trainers guide clients in analyzing triggers and extracting lessons instead of labeling the experience as failure. Encouraging reflection and resilience reinforces long-term commitment. Effective coaches frame each obstacle as an opportunity for learning, promoting emotional regulation and adaptability. Through this mindset, clients develop the psychological endurance needed to sustain progress across the inevitable fluctuations of real life.

Cultural Sensitivity and Individual Differences

Every client brings unique cultural, social, and personal perspectives to the training relationship. Cultural sensitivity acknowledges these differences, ensuring that communication, goal setting, and motivational strategies are respectful and inclusive. Trainers must avoid assumptions about values, diet, or exercise preferences based on background or appearance. Instead, they should ask open, curious questions about each client's experiences and traditions. Awareness of language nuances and nonverbal cues enhances understanding, especially across diverse populations. Cultural competence also includes accessibility—recognizing potential financial, physical, or environmental limitations that influence participation. Inclusive coaching fosters belonging, which strengthens adherence and trust. The culturally aware trainer adapts—not dilutes—their methods to reflect the client's reality. By embracing diversity as an asset rather than an obstacle, professionals create environments where all individuals feel seen, respected, and motivated to pursue health on their own terms.

Emotional Intelligence and Coaching Presence

Emotional intelligence is the ability to perceive, understand, and regulate emotions in oneself and others. In coaching, it distinguishes technical competence from transformative influence. Trainers with high emotional intelligence recognize subtle shifts in tone, posture, or expression, adjusting their approach accordingly. Self-awareness allows the coach to manage personal reactions, maintaining composure under stress. Empathy facilitates connection, while social awareness guides timing and tone of feedback. Coaching presence—the capacity to be fully attentive and engaged—amplifies emotional intelligence in action. It means being mentally available, listening beyond data, and responding authentically. This presence transforms each interaction into a moment of trust and insight. Emotionally intelligent trainers inspire confidence not through authority but through understanding. They cultivate environments where clients feel capable, valued, and motivated. Ultimately, emotional intelligence anchors behavioral coaching in humanity, reminding both trainer and client that sustainable change begins with compassion and mindful awareness.

Chapter 7: Professional Development and Responsibility

The Evolution of the Fitness Profession

The fitness industry has transformed from informal exercise instruction into a structured, science-based profession governed by ethics, certification, and continuing education. This evolution reflects society's growing recognition of health as a lifelong pursuit rather than a temporary goal. Certified personal trainers now serve as frontline health professionals, bridging preventive medicine and performance enhancement. The profession demands technical knowledge, emotional intelligence, and a commitment to evidence-based practice. As standards evolve, trainers must remain adaptable—embracing new research, technology, and interdisciplinary collaboration. Professional identity is not defined solely by certification but by conduct, consistency, and the ability to foster trust. Trainers represent the credibility of the industry; therefore, professionalism must be demonstrated in every interaction, from first consultation to final session. The modern trainer stands as both educator and role model, promoting not only physical improvement but also holistic well-being. The profession's credibility depends on those who uphold its scientific foundation and ethical integrity.

Scope of Practice and Professional Boundaries

Understanding and respecting the scope of practice defines professional responsibility. The certified trainer operates within clear parameters—designing and instructing safe, effective exercise programs while avoiding medical diagnosis, prescription, or therapy. Trainers collaborate with allied health professionals such as physicians, physical therapists, and dietitians when a client's needs exceed their qualifications. Staying within scope preserves both client safety and professional credibility. The trainer's authority lies in education, not medical intervention; recognizing this distinction prevents legal and ethical violations. Boundaries extend beyond expertise—they also include emotional and personal limits. Professional relationships must remain structured and goal-oriented, avoiding dependency or dual roles. Adhering to the scope of practice demonstrates respect for clients and the broader health community. Trainers who communicate openly about limitations not only protect themselves but also enhance trust, positioning fitness as an integral yet clearly defined component of comprehensive health care.

Ethics, Integrity, and Professional Conduct

Ethics in fitness transcend compliance; they embody a commitment to honesty, fairness, and respect for human dignity. Integrity guides every professional decision—from marketing claims to data confidentiality. Trainers must communicate truthfully about qualifications, avoid exaggerated promises, and ensure informed consent before assessments or interventions. Confidentiality protects client privacy, while non-discrimination ensures inclusivity regardless of age, gender, or background. Ethical practice also involves transparent billing, responsible referrals, and accountability for outcomes. When confronted with dilemmas, professionals rely on ethical reasoning frameworks—balancing client welfare, professional duty, and societal responsibility. Integrity is revealed not in public recognition but in consistent, unseen actions that build trust over time. Adherence to ethical codes, such as those outlined by NASM and ACSM, reinforces professionalism across the entire industry. Ethical trainers set the standard for excellence, proving that credibility arises not merely from knowledge but from moral character and reliability.

Legal Responsibilities and Risk Management

Legal literacy safeguards both clients and professionals. Trainers operate within environments that carry inherent physical risk, making proactive risk management essential. Understanding legal concepts—such as negligence, duty of care, and informed consent—prevents potential liability. Every client interaction should begin with a thorough screening process and signed documentation acknowledging program participation and associated risks. Proper supervision, equipment maintenance, and adherence to safety guidelines reduce exposure to claims of negligence. Record-keeping provides objective evidence of professional diligence, particularly in cases of incident review. Trainers should also maintain professional liability insurance as an essential safeguard. Beyond legal compliance, risk management reflects ethical care; it demonstrates foresight and respect for client welfare. A legally aware trainer views documentation not as bureaucracy but as protection for both parties. Through preparation and prudence, fitness professionals create environments of trust, safety, and professionalism, fulfilling their responsibility to operate with competence and accountability.

Continuing Education and Lifelong Learning

The hallmark of professionalism is an enduring commitment to education. The science of exercise evolves rapidly, demanding that trainers remain informed of new evidence, methodologies, and technologies. Continuing education ensures relevance, reinforces safety, and enhances credibility. Certifications require renewal precisely to promote this ongoing learning process. Trainers should pursue advanced courses, workshops, and research updates that broaden expertise beyond the minimum standard. Learning is not limited to technical knowledge—it includes emotional intelligence, business acumen, and communication skills. Reflective practice, mentorship, and peer collaboration further enrich professional growth. Lifelong learning transforms the trainer into a dynamic professional capable of adapting to emerging challenges. It embodies humility—the recognition that mastery is not a destination but a process. By continuously refining their craft, trainers maintain excellence, inspire confidence, and contribute to the collective advancement of the fitness profession.

Business Management and Professional Branding

Success in fitness extends beyond scientific knowledge to include business proficiency. Trainers operate within a service-based industry that demands effective management of time, finances, and reputation. Professional branding begins with clarity of purpose and authenticity—communicating expertise through consistent language, imagery, and behavior. Ethical marketing avoids exaggeration or unrealistic claims, focusing instead on transparency and value. Financial literacy supports sustainability through proper pricing, budgeting, and record-keeping. Client retention depends as much on business ethics as on exercise outcomes; professionalism, punctuality, and clear communication distinguish respected practitioners. Trainers may function independently or within organizations, but in either case, business integrity reflects professional identity. Strategic branding, informed by genuine expertise and credibility, positions the trainer as a trusted authority rather than a salesperson. Mastery of business operations ensures not only personal success but also the continued growth and respectability of the fitness industry as a whole.

Interdisciplinary Collaboration and Referral Networks

Modern health and fitness operate as parts of a larger continuum of care. Collaboration with healthcare professionals ensures comprehensive support for clients. Trainers should maintain referral networks that include physicians, registered dietitians, physical therapists, and mental health specialists. Recognizing when to refer is a sign of professionalism, not weakness. Interdisciplinary cooperation enhances program safety and effectiveness by integrating expertise from multiple disciplines. For example, a trainer may work alongside a physiotherapist to adapt post-rehabilitation exercises or coordinate with a nutritionist for dietary planning. Communication within these networks must remain concise, respectful, and client-centered. Documentation of referrals and feedback loops ensures continuity of care. Collaborative professionalism also elevates the industry's credibility within the healthcare community. By functioning as a bridge rather than a silo, the personal trainer contributes to a holistic model of health promotion that extends far beyond the gym.

Cultural and Ethical Inclusivity in Practice

Inclusive practice acknowledges that health and fitness are universal rights, not privileges. Trainers must ensure accessibility, respect for diversity, and cultural sensitivity in all client interactions. This includes awareness of socioeconomic, religious, gender, and ability-related factors that shape attitudes toward exercise. Ethical inclusivity requires more than tolerance—it demands active adaptation of communication, program design, and facility environment to meet diverse needs. Trainers should use language that affirms rather than excludes and remain open to learning from clients' lived experiences. Accessibility also encompasses physical space and financial options, ensuring that barriers to participation are minimized. Ethical inclusivity strengthens rapport, promotes equity, and aligns with the moral purpose of the profession: improving quality of life for all. Through respect and flexibility, trainers cultivate environments where every individual feels valued, safe, and empowered to pursue health on their own terms.

Professional Networking and Career Growth

Networking serves as a catalyst for opportunity and development. Building professional relationships with peers, mentors, and industry organizations expands knowledge and visibility. Conferences, workshops, and online forums allow trainers to share insights, exchange feedback, and stay abreast of emerging trends. Effective networking is based on authenticity, reciprocity, and professionalism—not self-promotion. A well-maintained professional network supports collaboration, referrals, and mentorship opportunities that enhance career longevity. Trainers should view networking as an extension of continuous education—an interactive process that strengthens both individual and collective advancement. Professional organizations such as NASM and ACSM offer structured avenues for connection through certifications, research dissemination, and advocacy. Active participation in these communities fosters identity within a respected professional body, transforming isolated practice into collaborative contribution. Networking, therefore, becomes not merely a career strategy but an ethical responsibility to elevate standards across the fitness profession.

Leadership and the Future of the Profession

Leadership within fitness extends beyond administrative authority—it represents the ability to inspire, guide, and uphold professional values. Trainers who model integrity, inclusivity, and evidence-based practice influence peers and clients alike. Leadership manifests in mentorship, community outreach, and advocacy for ethical standards. As technology reshapes fitness delivery through virtual platforms and data analytics, leaders must balance innovation with human connection. The future of the profession depends on educators and practitioners who champion credibility, accessibility, and lifelong learning. By mentoring new trainers and contributing to public health initiatives, professionals strengthen the link between fitness and preventive medicine. True leadership in fitness is quiet yet powerful—it uplifts others, protects ethical practice, and ensures that the industry evolves with both scientific precision and compassionate purpose.

Chapter 8 – Practice Questions

Questions (1-100)

Q1. Which part of a neuron transmits electrical impulses away from the cell body?
A. Dendrite
B. Soma
C. Axon
D. Synapse

Q2. During an eccentric contraction, what happens to the muscle fibers?
A. They shorten while producing tension
B. They lengthen while producing tension
C. They remain static with constant tension
D. They relax completely

Q3. Which system is primarily responsible for delivering oxygen and nutrients to working muscles during exercise?
A. Endocrine system
B. Nervous system
C. Cardiorespiratory system
D. Skeletal system

Q4. A client experiences a rapid increase in breathing rate during high-intensity training. Which physiological system is most involved?
A. Endocrine
B. Respiratory
C. Nervous
D. Digestive

Q5. What energy system provides the majority of ATP during the first 10 seconds of sprinting?
A. Glycolytic system
B. ATP–PC system
C. Oxidative system
D. Electron transport chain

Q6. Which structure connects muscle to bone?
A. Tendon
B. Ligament
C. Fascia
D. Cartilage

Q7. What is the main function of the synovial fluid found in joints?
A. Provides oxygen to ligaments
B. Prevents bone remodeling
C. Reduces friction and nourishes cartilage
D. Strengthens tendon attachment

Q8. Which plane of motion divides the body into right and left halves?
A. Frontal
B. Sagittal
C. Transverse
D. Coronal

Q9. What hormone increases heart rate and prepares the body for physical activity?

A. Cortisol
B. Insulin
C. Epinephrine
D. Testosterone

Q10. Which of the following best describes motor learning?
A. Short-term changes in muscle strength
B. Acquiring and refining movement skills through practice
C. Structural adaptation of muscle fibers
D. Immediate neural reflex response

Q11. Which type of muscle fiber has the greatest oxidative capacity and fatigue resistance?
A. Type IIx
B. Type IIa
C. Type I
D. Type IIb

Q12. What is the primary function of the cerebellum during movement?
A. Generating voluntary movement
B. Managing sensory input only
C. Regulating hormone secretion
D. Coordinating balance and motor control

Q13. Which connective tissue layer surrounds individual muscle fibers?
A. Epimysium
B. Perimysium
C. Endomysium
D. Sarcolemma

Q14. During aerobic exercise, what is the main energy substrate used after approximately 20 minutes?
A. Creatine phosphate
B. Glycogen
C. Fatty acids
D. Amino acids

Q15. Which term describes the body's ability to maintain a stable internal environment?
A. Allostasis
B. Metabolism
C. Homeostasis
D. Thermogenesis

Q16. Which muscle group is primarily responsible for extending the knee?
A. Hamstrings
B. Quadriceps
C. Gastrocnemius
D. Gluteals

Q17. What is the functional unit of a muscle fiber?
A. Sarcomere
B. Myofibril
C. Myosin
D. Fascicle

Q18. Which organ system helps regulate body temperature through sweat production?
A. Muscular
B. Integumentary
C. Endocrine

D. Circulatory

Q19. Which energy system provides ATP predominantly during long-duration, low-intensity exercise?

A. Phosphagen
B. Glycolytic
C. Oxidative
D. Lactic

Q20. What part of the brain initiates voluntary movement?

A. Medulla oblongata
B. Cerebellum
C. Motor cortex
D. Pons

Q21. A personal trainer notes a client's elevated resting heart rate. Which system is likely overactive?

A. Parasympathetic nervous system
B. Sympathetic nervous system
C. Somatic nervous system
D. Endocrine system

Q22. Which molecule directly supplies energy for muscle contraction?

A. Glucose
B. ATP
C. Creatine
D. Pyruvate

Q23. Which of the following is an example of an isometric exercise?

A. Bicep curl
B. Push-up
C. Squat jump
D. Wall sit

Q24. What is the role of mitochondria in muscle cells?

A. Store calcium ions for contraction
B. Generate ATP through aerobic metabolism
C. Produce lactic acid during exercise
D. Initiate nerve impulses

Q25. Which type of lever system is most common in the human body?

A. First-class
B. Second-class
C. Third-class
D. Fourth-class

Q26. What is the primary function of the nervous system in human movement?

A. Producing hormones for energy regulation
B. Coordinating and controlling all bodily actions
C. Transporting oxygen to working muscles
D. Maintaining bone mineral density

Q27. Which type of joint allows movement in all three planes?

A. Hinge joint
B. Pivot joint
C. Ball-and-socket joint
D. Saddle joint

Q28. During exercise, what is the main purpose of increased cardiac output?

A. Reducing core temperature

B. Supplying more oxygen and nutrients to muscles
C. Enhancing digestion rate
D. Slowing metabolic activity

Q29. Which metabolic pathway primarily uses glucose without oxygen to generate ATP?
A. Oxidative phosphorylation
B. ATP–PC system
C. Anaerobic glycolysis
D. Beta oxidation

Q30. What is the main function of red blood cells during exercise?
A. Transport oxygen and carbon dioxide
B. Regulate body temperature
C. Produce hormones for muscle growth
D. Maintain electrolyte balance

Q31. What is the role of calcium ions in muscle contraction?
A. Provide energy for the sliding filament action
B. Bind to troponin to expose actin-binding sites
C. Break down ATP for force production
D. Transmit nerve impulses across the synapse

Q32. Which muscle acts as the prime mover during a biceps curl?
A. Triceps brachii
B. Deltoid
C. Biceps brachii
D. Brachioradialis

Q33. Which term describes the relationship where a muscle shortens as it overcomes resistance?
A. Isometric
B. Isotonic concentric
C. Isotonic eccentric
D. Isokinetic

Q34. What organ controls the release of most hormones in the endocrine system?
A. Thyroid gland
B. Pituitary gland
C. Pancreas
D. Adrenal gland

Q35. During exercise, which hormone primarily increases glucose availability for working muscles?
A. Insulin
B. Cortisol
C. Epinephrine
D. Glucagon

Q36. What is the term for the smallest structural and functional unit of the nervous system?
A. Brainstem
B. Neuron
C. Synapse
D. Axon

Q37. During inhalation, which muscle primarily contracts to expand the thoracic cavity?
A. Diaphragm
B. Rectus abdominis
C. Pectoralis major
D. External oblique

Q38. Which principle explains that energy cannot be created or destroyed but only transformed?
A. Principle of overload
B. Law of thermodynamics
C. Principle of specificity
D. Law of adaptation
Q39. Which type of muscle fiber is best suited for short, explosive power activities?
A. Type I
B. Type IIa
C. Type IIx
D. Type I oxidative
Q40. Which feedback mechanism maintains homeostasis by reversing a physiological change?
A. Negative feedback
B. Positive feedback
C. Reciprocal inhibition
D. Reflex arc
Q41. Which structure allows communication between neurons?
A. Axon terminal
B. Synapse
C. Dendrite
D. Soma
Q42. Which system regulates long-term processes such as growth, metabolism, and reproduction?
A. Nervous system
B. Muscular system
C. Endocrine system
D. Circulatory system
Q43. What is the primary purpose of proprioceptors within muscles and joints?
A. Detect blood flow changes
B. Monitor body position and movement
C. Regulate hormone secretion
D. Control sweat production
Q44. Which metabolic pathway produces the highest ATP yield per molecule of glucose?
A. Anaerobic glycolysis
B. ATP–PC system
C. Aerobic respiration
D. Lactic acid pathway
Q45. What structure within skeletal muscle stores calcium necessary for contraction?
A. Myofibril
B. Sarcoplasmic reticulum
C. Sarcolemma
D. Mitochondria
Q46. Which process describes the body's ability to adapt to repeated exercise stimuli?
A. Overtraining
B. Homeostasis
C. General adaptation
D. Periodization
Q47. Which structure in the brain helps maintain vital functions such as heart rate and breathing?
A. Cerebrum
B. Cerebellum

C. Hypothalamus
D. Medulla oblongata

Q48. Which of the following represents an antagonistic muscle pair?
A. Quadriceps and hamstrings
B. Biceps and deltoids
C. Gluteals and abdominals
D. Trapezius and pectorals

Q49. What is the primary function of the skeletal system during physical activity?
A. Hormone synthesis
B. Energy production
C. Structural support and movement leverage
D. Oxygen storage

Q50. What is the role of ATP synthase during aerobic metabolism?
A. Transports electrons in the Krebs cycle
B. Regenerates ATP using energy from hydrogen ions
C. Breaks down glucose into pyruvate
D. Converts lactic acid to glycogen

Q51. What is the primary role of the mitochondria during exercise?
A. Store calcium for contraction
B. Produce ATP via aerobic metabolism
C. Generate lactic acid
D. Transmit nerve impulses

Q52. Which muscle fiber type is primarily activated during marathon running?
A. Type IIx
B. Type IIa
C. Type I
D. Type IIB

Q53. Which muscle is responsible for plantar flexion at the ankle joint?
A. Tibialis anterior
B. Gastrocnemius
C. Quadriceps
D. Sartorius

Q54. Which process allows oxygen and carbon dioxide exchange between the lungs and blood?
A. Filtration
B. Diffusion
C. Osmosis
D. Active transport

Q55. What structure detects changes in muscle tension to prevent injury?
A. Muscle spindle
B. Golgi tendon organ
C. Joint capsule
D. Ruffini ending

Q56. Which molecule is formed at the end of glycolysis before entering the Krebs cycle?
A. Acetyl-CoA
B. Citrate
C. Lactate
D. Pyruvate

Q57. What is the main purpose of the cardiovascular system during physical activity?

A. Distribute neural impulses
B. Deliver oxygen and nutrients while removing wastes
C. Maintain bone mineral density
D. Store glycogen for future use

Q58. Which energy system dominates during a 400-meter sprint lasting about 60 seconds?
A. ATP–PC system
B. Anaerobic glycolysis
C. Oxidative phosphorylation
D. Beta oxidation

Q59. Which joint movement decreases the angle between two bones?
A. Extension
B. Rotation
C. Flexion
D. Abduction

Q60. What is the function of myosin in muscle contraction?
A. Stores calcium
B. Forms the thin filament
C. Provides cross-bridges that pull actin filaments
D. Regulates neuromuscular junction

Q61. Which muscle acts as a stabilizer during a bench press?
A. Rotator cuff
B. Pectoralis major
C. Triceps brachii
D. Biceps brachii

Q62. During exercise, which mechanism helps maintain blood glucose levels?
A. Increased insulin secretion
B. Decreased glucagon secretion
C. Increased glycogen breakdown in the liver
D. Reduced cortisol levels

Q63. What is the primary function of ATP within the cell?
A. Acts as an enzyme for metabolism
B. Provides immediate energy for biological work
C. Stores oxygen for mitochondrial use
D. Transports nutrients across membranes

Q64. Which type of muscle contraction occurs when tension is produced without changing muscle length?
A. Isometric
B. Concentric
C. Eccentric
D. Plyometric

Q65. What part of the heart pumps oxygenated blood to the body?
A. Right atrium
B. Left atrium
C. Right ventricle
D. Left ventricle

Q66. Which structure detects muscle length and rate of stretch?
A. Golgi tendon organ
B. Muscle spindle

C. Pacinian corpuscle
D. Free nerve ending

Q67. What process converts fatty acids into acetyl-CoA for entry into the Krebs cycle?
A. Glycolysis
B. Beta oxidation
C. Deamination
D. Transamination

Q68. What happens to stroke volume as exercise intensity increases?
A. It decreases
B. It remains constant
C. It increases then plateaus
D. It continuously rises linearly

Q69. Which muscle group stabilizes the spine during lifting exercises?
A. Rectus abdominis
B. Erector spinae
C. Hip flexors
D. Latissimus dorsi

Q70. Which mechanism initiates muscle contraction after nerve stimulation?
A. Calcium release from sarcoplasmic reticulum
B. ATP breakdown into ADP
C. Myosin head detachment
D. Sodium reuptake into neurons

Q71. What is the primary function of hemoglobin?
A. Transport oxygen in the blood
B. Control blood pH
C. Aid in digestion
D. Act as an enzyme

Q72. Which factor primarily determines the intensity of aerobic metabolism during exercise?
A. ATP concentration
B. Oxygen availability
C. Lactic acid buildup
D. Core temperature

Q73. Which part of the neuron receives incoming signals from other neurons?
A. Axon
B. Dendrite
C. Soma
D. Synaptic cleft

Q74. What structure anchors the actin filaments within the sarcomere?
A. M line
B. H zone
C. Z line
D. A band

Q75. Which of the following represents the body's immediate energy source during muscular contraction?
A. Creatine phosphate
B. Glycogen
C. Fatty acids
D. Lactic acid

Q76. Which term describes the process of converting non-carbohydrate sources like amino acids into glucose?
A. Glycogenolysis
B. Gluconeogenesis
C. Glycolysis
D. Lipolysis
Q77. What is the primary role of the Krebs cycle in energy production?
A. To synthesize glycogen
B. To create lactic acid for anaerobic metabolism
C. To store ATP in the muscle
D. To oxidize acetyl-CoA and generate NADH and $FADH_2$
Q78. Which organ plays the most significant role in maintaining blood pH during exercise?
A. Liver
B. Kidneys
C. Lungs
D. Pancreas
Q79. During resistance training, what stimulates muscle hypertrophy the most?
A. Low mechanical tension
B. Short rest periods only
C. High mechanical tension and progressive overload
D. Minimal muscle activation
Q80. Which type of skeletal muscle fiber has moderate fatigue resistance and both aerobic and anaerobic capacity?
A. Type I
B. Type IIa
C. Type IIx
D. Type IIB
Q81. Which system is directly responsible for controlling heart rate during exercise?
A. Autonomic nervous system
B. Somatic nervous system
C. Endocrine system
D. Central nervous system only
Q82. What is the primary byproduct of anaerobic glycolysis when oxygen is limited?
A. Carbon dioxide
B. Lactate
C. Pyruvate
D. Acetyl-CoA
Q83. Which part of the respiratory system is responsible for gas exchange?
A. Trachea
B. Bronchi
C. Alveoli
D. Diaphragm
Q84. Which hormone facilitates glucose uptake into cells after meals?
A. Insulin
B. Cortisol
C. Epinephrine
D. Glucagon
Q85. What is the effect of chronic endurance training on resting heart rate?

A. It increases
B. It decreases
C. It fluctuates randomly
D. It remains unchanged

Q86. What happens to blood pressure during aerobic exercise?
A. Both systolic and diastolic pressure decrease
B. Systolic pressure increases, diastolic remains stable or decreases slightly
C. Both pressures rise sharply
D. Diastolic pressure increases significantly

Q87. What is the role of creatine phosphate in the ATP–PC system?
A. To store glucose for later use
B. To transport oxygen to muscles
C. To produce lactic acid for energy
D. To provide phosphate for rapid ATP regeneration

Q88. What is the primary function of the cerebrum in movement?
A. Controls automatic breathing
B. Coordinates fine motor skills and voluntary actions
C. Maintains balance and posture reflexes
D. Regulates hormone secretion

Q89. Which electrolyte is most critical for generating muscle action potentials?
A. Calcium
B. Potassium
C. Sodium
D. Magnesium

Q90. What physiological response occurs to improve oxygen delivery during high-intensity exercise?
A. Decreased ventilation rate
B. Increased heart rate and stroke volume
C. Reduced cardiac output
D. Lowered arterial pressure

Q91. Which form should always be completed before conducting any fitness assessments with a new client?
A. Health history questionnaire
B. PAR-Q (Physical Activity Readiness Questionnaire)
C. Informed consent form
D. Waiver of liability

Q92. A client's resting heart rate is measured at 92 bpm. What does this indicate?
A. Normal range for a healthy adult
B. Bradycardia
C. Elevated resting heart rate
D. Excellent cardiovascular conditioning

Q93. What is the primary purpose of the overhead squat assessment?
A. Evaluate cardiovascular endurance
B. Identify movement compensations and postural imbalances
C. Measure lower-body strength
D. Assess flexibility only

Q94. Which of the following is an example of a subjective assessment?
A. Blood pressure reading
B. Resting heart rate

C. Client's occupation and stress level
D. Body fat percentage

Q95. A personal trainer observes excessive forward lean during an overhead squat. Which muscle is most likely overactive?

A. Anterior tibialis
B. Gluteus maximus
C. Soleus
D. Erector spinae

Q96. What is the recommended time for measuring a client's resting heart rate?

A. Immediately after waking up
B. After a workout
C. Midday after lunch
D. Before bedtime

Q97. Which assessment best evaluates upper-body pushing movement patterns?

A. Push-up test
B. Overhead squat test
C. Rockport walk test
D. Step-up test

Q98. During postural assessment, a client shows rounded shoulders. Which muscle is most likely overactive?

A. Middle trapezius
B. Rhomboids
C. Pectoralis major
D. Posterior deltoid

Q99. Which test is used to measure lower-body muscular strength?

A. Push-up test
B. Bench press test
C. YMCA step test
D. Squat strength assessment (1RM)

Q100. Which assessment evaluates cardiorespiratory endurance in deconditioned clients?

A. Rockport Walk Test
B. 1.5-Mile Run Test
C. Step-Up Test
D. Cooper 12-Minute Run

Answer keys and Explanations (1-100)

Q1. Answer: C

Explanation: The axon conducts electrical impulses away from the neuron's cell body toward other neurons or muscles. This transmission occurs via action potentials that travel along the axon membrane. Myelination increases the speed of impulse conduction, allowing rapid communication between the nervous system and muscle tissue necessary for coordinated movement.

Q2. Answer: B

Explanation: In eccentric contractions, muscle fibers lengthen while still generating tension to control movement or resist external force. This controlled lengthening allows smooth deceleration and stabilization of joints during activities such as lowering a weight or landing from a jump, making it crucial for functional strength and injury prevention.

Q3. Answer: C

Explanation: The cardiorespiratory system, composed of the heart, blood vessels, and lungs, delivers oxygen and nutrients while removing waste like carbon dioxide. This system's efficiency directly influences exercise performance and endurance, as improved oxygen delivery supports sustained ATP production through aerobic metabolism.

Q4. Answer: B

Explanation: The respiratory system adjusts ventilation rate during exercise to meet increased oxygen demands and expel excess carbon dioxide. This physiological response maintains acid-base balance and supports cellular metabolism, ensuring muscles receive adequate oxygen to sustain energy production during exertion.

Q5. Answer: B

Explanation: The ATP–PC system (phosphagen system) dominates during short, high-intensity efforts by breaking down phosphocreatine to regenerate ATP rapidly. Although it provides energy quickly, this system depletes within about 10 seconds, after which the glycolytic pathway becomes more active to sustain performance.

Q6. Answer: A

Explanation: Tendons are dense connective tissues that transmit force generated by muscle contraction to bones, enabling movement. Their strong collagen composition allows them to withstand tension, making them essential for stability and motion efficiency during exercise and everyday activities.

Q7. Answer: C

Explanation: Synovial fluid acts as a lubricant, minimizing friction between articulating bones, while also nourishing and maintaining cartilage health. This fluid ensures smooth, pain-free joint movement, which is crucial for maintaining flexibility and preventing wear during repetitive or dynamic exercise.

Q8. Answer: B

Explanation: The sagittal plane divides the body into right and left sides, allowing movements such as flexion and extension. Understanding planes of motion helps trainers design balanced programs addressing all movement directions to improve functional performance and prevent muscular imbalances.

Q9. Answer: C

Explanation: Epinephrine, also known as adrenaline, is secreted by the adrenal medulla and stimulates increased heart rate, respiratory rate, and energy availability. This hormone activates the "fight-or-flight" response, enhancing oxygen and nutrient delivery to muscles during intense exercise.

Q10. Answer: B

Explanation: Motor learning is the process of acquiring and improving movement efficiency through repeated practice and feedback. This adaptation leads to better coordination and precision, allowing consistent execution of exercises and enhanced athletic performance over time.

Q11. Answer: C

Explanation: Type I (slow-twitch) fibers rely primarily on aerobic metabolism, contain abundant mitochondria, and have rich capillary networks. These characteristics allow them to sustain low-intensity, endurance activities such as jogging or cycling for long periods without fatigue.

Q12. Answer: D

Explanation: The cerebellum refines motor commands from the brain, ensuring smooth, coordinated, and balanced movements. It integrates sensory feedback from muscles and joints to adjust motion accuracy, playing a vital role in posture and exercise technique precision.

Q13. Answer: C

Explanation: The endomysium is a thin connective tissue layer enveloping each muscle fiber, providing structural integrity and enabling transmission of force within the muscle. It also contains capillaries and nerves that supply each fiber with nutrients and signals for contraction.

Q14. Answer: C

Explanation: After prolonged moderate-intensity exercise, the body increasingly relies on fatty acids for ATP production as glycogen stores diminish. This shift toward fat metabolism enhances endurance efficiency, allowing extended performance without rapid fatigue or energy depletion.

Q15. Answer: C

Explanation: Homeostasis is the body's mechanism to preserve internal balance—such as temperature, pH, and fluid levels—despite external stressors. Exercise challenges homeostasis, prompting adaptations that improve physiological efficiency and resilience to future physical demands.

Q16. Answer: B

Explanation: The quadriceps femoris group, located on the front of the thigh, extends the knee joint. This powerful muscle group is essential for movements such as squatting, jumping, and running, providing propulsion and stability during dynamic activities.

Q17. Answer: A

Explanation: The sarcomere is the smallest functional unit of muscle contraction, composed of actin and myosin filaments. Its repeated structure along myofibrils generates tension through the sliding filament mechanism, enabling controlled and powerful muscle contractions.

Q18. Answer: B

Explanation: The integumentary system, particularly sweat glands in the skin, aids thermoregulation by releasing sweat to dissipate heat. This mechanism prevents overheating during exercise, maintaining performance efficiency and protecting vital organs.

Q19. Answer: C

Explanation: The oxidative (aerobic) system sustains ATP production during prolonged activities by metabolizing carbohydrates and fats with oxygen. This efficient process supports endurance performance, allowing athletes to maintain steady effort over extended periods.

Q20. Answer: C

Explanation: The motor cortex in the frontal lobe sends neural signals through descending pathways to skeletal muscles, initiating voluntary movement. This region is essential for controlled exercise execution and development of motor patterns.

Q21. Answer: B

Explanation: The sympathetic nervous system activates during stress or exertion, increasing heart rate and energy mobilization. Chronic overactivation can elevate resting heart rate and fatigue levels, highlighting the importance of recovery and stress management.

Q22. Answer: B

Explanation: Adenosine triphosphate (ATP) provides the immediate energy required for muscle contraction. When ATP is hydrolyzed to ADP and phosphate, energy is released to power the sliding of actin and myosin filaments, enabling movement.

Q23. Answer: D

Explanation: A wall sit involves generating tension without joint movement, classifying it as an isometric exercise. This static contraction improves muscular endurance and stabilization by recruiting postural muscles to maintain a fixed position under load.

Q24. Answer: B

Explanation: Mitochondria are the cell's powerhouses, converting oxygen and nutrients into ATP via oxidative phosphorylation. Increased mitochondrial density enhances endurance capacity by improving muscles' ability to sustain prolonged aerobic activity.

Q25. Answer: C

Explanation: Most human movements operate as third-class levers, where the effort is applied between the fulcrum and the load. This design prioritizes speed and range of motion, allowing efficient, rapid limb movements essential for athletic and daily tasks.

Q26. Answer: B

Explanation: The nervous system acts as the command center of the body, coordinating and controlling all movement and physiological responses. It transmits electrical impulses that signal muscles to contract, adjust posture, and respond to external stimuli. This communication between the brain, spinal cord, and peripheral nerves ensures precise timing, efficiency, and control of voluntary and involuntary movements during exercise and daily activity.

Q27. Answer: C

Explanation: A ball-and-socket joint, like the shoulder or hip, permits movement in all three planes—sagittal, frontal, and transverse—providing the greatest range of motion. Its spherical head fits into a cup-shaped cavity, allowing flexion, extension, abduction, adduction, and rotation. This multi-directional mobility is vital for complex athletic movements such as throwing, swimming, and dancing, but requires strong muscular stabilization for joint protection.

Q28. Answer: B

Explanation: Cardiac output rises during exercise to meet muscles' elevated oxygen and nutrient demands. The heart pumps more blood per minute by increasing stroke volume and heart rate, ensuring efficient oxygen delivery and waste removal. This enhanced circulation supports sustained energy production through aerobic metabolism, enabling prolonged activity and delaying fatigue in both endurance and resistance training contexts.

Q29. Answer: C

Explanation: Anaerobic glycolysis rapidly converts glucose into ATP without requiring oxygen, producing lactate as a byproduct. This pathway is dominant during moderate-to-high intensity efforts lasting up to about two minutes, such as sprinting or circuit training. It provides a quick energy supply when oxygen delivery is limited, allowing continued muscle contraction despite the buildup of metabolic byproducts.

Q30. Answer: A

Explanation: Red blood cells contain hemoglobin, a protein that binds oxygen in the lungs and transports it to tissues while carrying carbon dioxide back for exhalation. During exercise, their oxygen delivery efficiency directly influences performance capacity. Enhanced red blood cell function supports greater aerobic endurance by optimizing oxygen availability for ATP production and delaying the onset of muscular fatigue.

Q31. Answer: B

Explanation: Calcium ions released from the sarcoplasmic reticulum bind to troponin, causing tropomyosin to shift and expose active sites on actin filaments. This allows myosin heads to attach and perform the power stroke that produces contraction. Calcium regulation ensures synchronized contraction and relaxation, making it a fundamental element in strength development and neuromuscular coordination during training.

Q32. Answer: C

Explanation: The biceps brachii serves as the prime mover, or agonist, in elbow flexion during a biceps curl. It generates the main force required to lift the load by contracting concentrically. This muscle's strength and endurance are crucial for upper-body pulling motions, and targeted training enhances grip strength, functional performance, and joint stability in everyday and athletic tasks.

Q33. Answer: B

Explanation: An isotonic concentric contraction occurs when a muscle shortens while producing force to overcome resistance. This action is typical in lifting movements like the upward phase of a biceps curl. Concentric training enhances power and strength by improving the muscle's ability to generate tension efficiently, which is fundamental in athletic performance and resistance-based programming.

Q34. Answer: B

Explanation: The pituitary gland, often called the "master gland," regulates hormone secretion from many other endocrine glands. It controls growth, metabolism, reproduction, and stress response by releasing stimulating hormones under hypothalamic direction. During exercise, it triggers hormonal cascades that influence energy availability, recovery, and tissue repair, making it essential for maintaining physiological balance and adaptation.

Q35. Answer: D

Explanation: Glucagon, secreted by the pancreas, promotes the breakdown of glycogen into glucose within the liver to maintain blood sugar levels during exercise. This process ensures continuous energy supply for active muscles when carbohydrate demand increases. Efficient glucagon response supports endurance and prevents hypoglycemia, particularly during prolonged or high-intensity training sessions.

Q36. Answer: B

Explanation: The neuron is the fundamental functional unit of the nervous system, responsible for transmitting electrical impulses. Each neuron consists of a cell body, dendrites, and an axon, allowing communication between the brain, spinal cord, and muscles. Neuronal efficiency is critical for motor control, reflex coordination, and quick muscular responses required in athletic performance and training adaptations.

Q37. Answer: A

Explanation: The diaphragm contracts and flattens during inhalation, increasing thoracic cavity volume and drawing air into the lungs. This muscle's rhythmic action supports oxygen delivery essential for aerobic metabolism. Training that improves diaphragmatic strength enhances respiratory efficiency, endurance, and overall performance during sustained physical activity.

Q38. Answer: B

Explanation: The first law of thermodynamics states that energy cannot be created or destroyed but transformed from one form to another. In exercise physiology, this means chemical energy from nutrients converts into mechanical energy for movement and heat. Understanding this concept underlies efficient energy system management, nutritional planning, and metabolic adaptation during training.

Q39. Answer: C

Explanation: Type IIx (fast-twitch) fibers generate high force and rapid contractions but fatigue quickly due to limited oxidative capacity. They rely heavily on anaerobic metabolism, making them ideal for sprinting, jumping, and resistance exercises requiring maximum intensity. Training that targets these fibers enhances power output, neuromuscular coordination, and overall athletic explosiveness.

Q40. Answer: A

Explanation: Negative feedback mechanisms restore equilibrium by counteracting deviations from normal physiological levels. For example, when body temperature rises, sweat production cools the body to maintain balance. This self-regulating process stabilizes internal conditions like blood pressure and glucose, allowing the body to function efficiently during exercise stress.

Q41. Answer: B

Explanation: The synapse is the junction where neurons communicate via chemical neurotransmitters or electrical signals. This process allows coordinated neural activity necessary for muscle activation, reflex responses, and movement control. Efficient synaptic transmission ensures rapid information processing, which supports smooth, precise physical performance in exercise and sports.

Q42. Answer: C

Explanation: The endocrine system releases hormones into the bloodstream to regulate prolonged bodily functions like growth, metabolism, and reproductive health. Unlike the rapid signaling of the nervous system, hormonal responses act more slowly but sustain longer effects. This regulation ensures energy balance, muscle repair, and physiological adaptation following exercise.

Q43. Answer: B

Explanation: Proprioceptors detect changes in muscle tension, joint angle, and body position, sending feedback to the nervous system. This sensory input helps coordinate posture, balance, and smooth motor activity during exercise. Enhanced proprioceptive function improves movement accuracy, reducing injury risk and supporting efficient technique execution.

Q44. Answer: C

Explanation: Aerobic respiration fully oxidizes glucose in the presence of oxygen through glycolysis, the Krebs cycle, and the electron transport chain, yielding about 36 ATP per glucose molecule. This efficient energy production supports prolonged, moderate-intensity exercise, allowing sustained muscle contraction without rapid fatigue.

Q45. Answer: B

Explanation: The sarcoplasmic reticulum stores and releases calcium ions upon neural stimulation, initiating the interaction between actin and myosin. Proper calcium handling enables smooth muscle contraction and relaxation cycles. Enhanced calcium regulation contributes to strength, endurance, and coordination during repetitive physical activity.

Q46. Answer: C

Explanation: General adaptation refers to the body's progressive physiological adjustments to repeated exercise stress. These adaptations—such as increased cardiovascular efficiency and muscular strength—occur through recovery and consistent training exposure. Understanding this process allows structured programming that enhances performance while minimizing the risk of overtraining.

Q47. Answer: D

Explanation: The medulla oblongata, located in the brainstem, regulates involuntary functions such as heart rate, respiration, and blood pressure. Its continuous control ensures survival and homeostasis, particularly under exercise stress when oxygen demand and cardiovascular activity increase significantly.

Q48. Answer: A

Explanation: The quadriceps and hamstrings act as antagonistic pairs—when one contracts, the other relaxes. This reciprocal coordination enables smooth joint motion and stability, essential for controlled limb movement during running, squatting, or jumping. Training both ensures balanced strength and reduces injury risk.

Q49. Answer: C

Explanation: The skeletal system provides a rigid framework that supports the body and serves as leverage for muscle attachment. Through joints and bones, it facilitates movement while protecting internal organs. Healthy skeletal structure ensures proper biomechanics and performance efficiency in exercise.

Q50. Answer: B

Explanation: ATP synthase, located in the mitochondria, synthesizes ATP by harnessing energy from hydrogen ion gradients generated during the electron transport chain. This enzyme is central to aerobic metabolism, providing a continuous energy supply for prolonged muscular activity and sustaining endurance performance.

Q51. Answer: B

Explanation: Mitochondria are the energy powerhouses of cells, responsible for producing ATP through aerobic metabolism. During prolonged exercise, they oxidize carbohydrates and fats to generate sustainable energy. Increased mitochondrial density enhances muscular endurance, delays fatigue, and supports recovery by improving the efficiency of oxygen utilization and ATP synthesis within skeletal muscle cells.

Q52. Answer: C

Explanation: Type I (slow-twitch) fibers are recruited during long-duration, low-intensity endurance activities like marathon running. They rely on aerobic metabolism, have a high mitochondrial content, and resist fatigue effectively. These fibers sustain energy output efficiently by using oxygen and fat as primary fuel sources, allowing consistent performance throughout prolonged exercise sessions.

Q53. Answer: B

Explanation: The gastrocnemius muscle, located in the posterior lower leg, performs plantar flexion—pointing the foot downward. It works synergistically with the soleus during walking, running, and jumping. Strengthening the gastrocnemius improves explosive lower-body performance, stability, and propulsion efficiency in dynamic athletic movements.

Q54. Answer: B

Explanation: Gas exchange occurs through diffusion, a passive process where oxygen moves from areas of higher concentration in the alveoli to lower concentration in the blood, while carbon dioxide moves oppositely. This exchange enables proper oxygen delivery to tissues and removal of waste gases, supporting cellular respiration during exercise.

Q55. Answer: B

Explanation: The Golgi tendon organ senses tension within tendons and triggers reflex inhibition when force becomes excessive, preventing muscle or tendon damage. This safety mechanism ensures controlled contraction and contributes to muscle coordination, particularly during heavy resistance training or high-force exertion activities.

Q56. Answer: D

Explanation: Glycolysis breaks down glucose into pyruvate, producing small amounts of ATP and NADH. In the presence of oxygen, pyruvate enters the mitochondria and is converted into acetyl-CoA, initiating the Krebs cycle for aerobic energy production. This process bridges anaerobic and aerobic pathways in cellular metabolism.

Q57. Answer: B

Explanation: The cardiovascular system ensures oxygen and nutrient delivery to active tissues while transporting metabolic byproducts like carbon dioxide and lactate away. Enhanced cardiac efficiency supports prolonged exercise capacity, faster recovery, and improved overall endurance through optimal blood circulation and tissue oxygenation.

Q58. Answer: B

Explanation: During a 400-meter sprint, anaerobic glycolysis predominates, breaking down glucose without oxygen to rapidly generate ATP. Though efficient short-term, this system produces lactic acid, leading to fatigue. Its role is crucial for high-intensity efforts lasting between 30 seconds and two minutes before aerobic pathways take over.

Q59. Answer: C

Explanation: Flexion occurs when the angle between two bones decreases, bringing the segments closer together. Common examples include bending the elbow or knee. Understanding flexion mechanics is essential for identifying movement planes and ensuring proper exercise form during resistance or flexibility training.

Q60. Answer: C

Explanation: Myosin constitutes the thick filament within a sarcomere and generates force by forming cross-bridges with actin filaments during contraction. The myosin heads pivot, pulling actin inward, shortening the muscle fiber. This power stroke cycle, fueled by ATP, produces movement and mechanical work during every muscular action.

Q61. Answer: A

Explanation: The rotator cuff muscles stabilize the shoulder joint during pressing movements, maintaining humeral head alignment within the socket. Their stabilizing function prevents excessive joint translation and supports efficient force transfer from prime movers like the pectoralis major and triceps, enhancing strength while minimizing injury risk.

Q62. Answer: C

Explanation: The liver breaks down stored glycogen into glucose, a process called glycogenolysis, to sustain blood glucose during exercise. This ensures continuous energy supply to muscles as demands rise. Hormones such as glucagon and epinephrine facilitate this mechanism, maintaining performance and preventing fatigue.

Q63. Answer: B

Explanation: ATP serves as the universal energy currency of the cell, fueling all metabolic reactions including muscle contraction, nerve impulse transmission, and biosynthesis. Hydrolysis of ATP releases energy that powers cellular processes essential for exercise performance and physiological maintenance.

Q64. Answer: A

Explanation: Isometric contractions generate force without altering muscle length or joint angle, maintaining static positions such as planks or wall sits. This contraction type enhances muscular endurance and stabilization, contributing to postural control and joint integrity during functional movement.

Q65. Answer: D

Explanation: The left ventricle's thick muscular walls generate strong contractions that propel oxygen-rich blood through the aorta to systemic circulation. Its powerful pumping capacity ensures adequate oxygen and nutrient distribution during exercise, supporting sustained muscle activity and performance.

Q66. Answer: B

Explanation: Muscle spindles monitor changes in muscle length and speed of stretch, triggering reflex contractions to prevent overstretching. This sensory feedback supports balance, coordination, and protective reflexes essential during dynamic exercise and flexibility training.

Q67. Answer: B

Explanation: Beta oxidation breaks down fatty acids into acetyl-CoA units within the mitochondria, enabling their entry into the Krebs cycle for aerobic energy production. This pathway predominates during prolonged, steady-state exercise when fat becomes a major fuel source.

Q68. Answer: C

Explanation: Stroke volume increases with exercise intensity due to greater venous return and myocardial contractility but plateaus at moderate levels in most individuals. Beyond that point, further cardiac output rises primarily through heart rate elevation, sustaining efficient blood flow during vigorous activity.

Q69. Answer: B

Explanation: The erector spinae muscles maintain spinal alignment and resist flexion during lifting movements. Their stabilizing role protects the vertebral column from excessive strain, allowing safe and efficient force transfer through the kinetic chain during resistance training.

Q70. Answer: A

Explanation: Nerve impulses trigger calcium release from the sarcoplasmic reticulum into the muscle cell cytoplasm. These ions bind to troponin, enabling cross-bridge formation between actin and myosin, which generates contraction. This precise calcium control ensures smooth, coordinated movement.

Q71. Answer: A

Explanation: Hemoglobin within red blood cells binds oxygen in the lungs and releases it to tissues where it's needed for metabolism. It also carries carbon dioxide back for exhalation. High hemoglobin levels enhance endurance by improving oxygen-carrying capacity.

Q72. Answer: B

Explanation: Oxygen availability dictates the rate of aerobic metabolism, as sufficient oxygen is necessary for oxidative phosphorylation within mitochondria. Higher oxygen delivery supports greater ATP production efficiency, allowing sustained energy output and endurance during extended exercise efforts.

Q73. Answer: B

Explanation: Dendrites are branched extensions that receive and conduct electrical signals toward the neuron's cell body. Their large surface area allows integration of multiple inputs, enabling complex coordination and sensory processing vital for motor control during physical movement.

Q74. Answer: C

Explanation: The Z line defines the sarcomere boundary and secures actin filaments, maintaining structural integrity during contraction. The distance between Z lines shortens as the muscle contracts, producing mechanical movement and force generation.

Q75. Answer: A

Explanation: Creatine phosphate rapidly donates a phosphate group to ADP to regenerate ATP, supplying immediate energy for high-intensity, short-duration efforts. This quick replenishment sustains explosive power output before slower energy systems activate.

Q76. Answer: B

Explanation: Gluconeogenesis occurs primarily in the liver, where amino acids, glycerol, and lactate are converted into glucose to maintain blood sugar during prolonged fasting or exercise. This process ensures a continuous energy supply when glycogen stores are depleted, supporting endurance and preventing hypoglycemia during extended physical activity or caloric restriction.

Q77. Answer: D

Explanation: The Krebs cycle, also known as the citric acid cycle, oxidizes acetyl-CoA derived from carbohydrates, fats, and proteins. It generates NADH and $FADH_2$, which carry high-energy electrons to the electron transport chain for ATP production. This central metabolic pathway supports sustained aerobic energy generation essential for endurance exercise.

Q78. Answer: C

Explanation: The lungs regulate blood pH during exercise by expelling carbon dioxide, a byproduct of metabolism that forms carbonic acid in the blood. Increased respiration removes CO_2, preventing acid buildup and maintaining acid-base balance. This buffering capacity ensures optimal enzyme function and delays fatigue during sustained effort.

Q79. Answer: C

Explanation: Muscle hypertrophy results primarily from sustained high mechanical tension combined with progressive overload, which triggers cellular signaling pathways that promote protein synthesis and muscle fiber growth. Consistent resistance training under these conditions increases cross-sectional muscle size, strength, and performance over time.

Q80. Answer: B

Explanation: Type IIa fibers are hybrid fast-twitch muscles that use both aerobic and anaerobic energy systems. They generate substantial power while maintaining reasonable endurance. This versatility allows them to adapt across training intensities, making them crucial for sports requiring repeated bursts of effort, such as soccer or basketball.

Q81. Answer: A

Explanation: The autonomic nervous system regulates involuntary functions like heart rate. During exercise, its sympathetic branch increases heart rate and cardiac output to meet oxygen demands, while the parasympathetic branch dominates during recovery to restore normal levels. This dynamic balance ensures efficient cardiovascular response and recovery.

Q82. Answer: B

Explanation: When oxygen is insufficient, pyruvate produced during glycolysis converts into lactate. This allows continued ATP generation under anaerobic conditions. Although lactate accumulation can temporarily reduce pH, it serves as a valuable energy source once oxygen levels normalize, supporting ongoing muscular activity and recovery.

Q83. Answer: C

Explanation: Alveoli are tiny air sacs in the lungs where oxygen diffuses into the bloodstream and carbon dioxide diffuses out. Their thin walls and extensive capillary networks maximize gas exchange efficiency. Healthy alveolar function is vital for maintaining aerobic capacity and endurance performance.

Q84. Answer: A

Explanation: Insulin, secreted by the pancreas, promotes glucose uptake into cells for immediate energy or glycogen storage. This hormone lowers blood sugar levels and supports energy replenishment post-exercise. Effective insulin function ensures proper nutrient utilization and recovery after physical activity.

Q85. Answer: B

Explanation: Regular endurance training enhances cardiac efficiency, leading to a lower resting heart rate. The heart pumps more blood per beat due to increased stroke volume, reducing the need for frequent contractions at rest. This adaptation reflects improved cardiovascular fitness and oxygen delivery efficiency.

Q86. Answer: B

Explanation: During aerobic exercise, systolic blood pressure rises to accommodate higher cardiac output, while diastolic pressure remains steady or slightly decreases due to vasodilation in active muscles. This controlled adjustment ensures adequate oxygen supply while maintaining vascular balance and preventing excessive strain on the circulatory system.

Q87. Answer: D

Explanation: Creatine phosphate donates a high-energy phosphate group to ADP, quickly regenerating ATP during short, explosive movements. This process supports immediate power output for 5–10 seconds of maximal effort, such as sprinting or weightlifting. Its efficiency makes it critical for high-intensity, anaerobic performance.

Q88. Answer: B

Explanation: The cerebrum, part of the forebrain, governs voluntary motor functions, conscious control, and precise coordination. It processes input from sensory systems and sends motor commands to execute movement. Efficient cerebrum activity enhances motor learning, coordination, and skill execution during exercise and sport performance.

Q89. Answer: C

Explanation: Sodium ions play a crucial role in initiating and transmitting muscle action potentials. When sodium channels open, positive ions flow into the cell, depolarizing the membrane and triggering contraction. Proper sodium balance supports nerve conduction and muscular responsiveness, preventing cramps or weakness during activity.

Q90. Answer: B

Explanation: During intense exercise, both heart rate and stroke volume increase, elevating cardiac output to deliver more oxygenated blood to working muscles. This enhanced circulatory response ensures sufficient oxygen transport for aerobic metabolism and energy production, sustaining performance and delaying fatigue.

Q91. Answer: B

Explanation: The PAR-Q identifies potential health risks and determines whether medical clearance is needed before physical activity. It helps ensure client safety by screening for cardiovascular, metabolic, or orthopedic conditions. Completing this form prior to testing protects both client and trainer while aligning with NASM's recommended pre-assessment protocols.

Q92. Answer: C

Explanation: A resting heart rate above 90 bpm is considered elevated and may suggest deconditioning, stress, or cardiovascular inefficiency. This information helps trainers monitor baseline fitness levels and tailor initial programming to emphasize aerobic conditioning and stress management techniques for improved heart rate regulation.

Q93. Answer: B

Explanation: The overhead squat assessment identifies movement dysfunctions and postural imbalances by evaluating dynamic flexibility, core stability, and neuromuscular control. Observing compensations during the squat reveals overactive and underactive muscles, allowing trainers to design corrective exercise strategies for improved movement efficiency and injury prevention.

Q94. Answer: C

Explanation: Subjective assessments involve client-reported information such as occupation, stress, and lifestyle habits. These insights provide context for movement patterns, energy levels, and potential barriers to exercise, guiding program customization. Unlike objective data, subjective inputs rely on personal perception and conversation.

Q95. Answer: C

Explanation: The soleus often contributes to excessive forward lean due to tightness restricting ankle dorsiflexion. This overactivity shifts the center of gravity forward, compromising squat mechanics. Corrective strategies typically include foam rolling and static stretching of the soleus while strengthening the anterior tibialis and gluteus maximus.

Q96. Answer: A

Explanation: Resting heart rate should be measured immediately after waking and before engaging in physical activity. This timing minimizes interference from stress, movement, or caffeine, ensuring an accurate reflection of cardiovascular baseline. Monitoring morning RHR over time helps track fitness improvements or signs of overtraining.

Q97. Answer: A

Explanation: The push-up test examines upper-body pushing mechanics and muscular endurance by engaging the chest, shoulders, and triceps. It also helps identify movement compensations such as low-back sag or shoulder elevation, providing insight into upper kinetic chain stability and strength imbalances.

Q98. Answer: C

Explanation: Overactivity in the pectoralis major and minor pulls the shoulders forward into protraction, leading to rounded posture. This imbalance often accompanies underactive upper-back muscles. Corrective training includes stretching the chest and strengthening the mid-trapezius, rhomboids, and posterior deltoids to restore alignment.

Q99. Answer: D

Explanation: The squat strength assessment (1RM) measures maximal lower-body force output, focusing on glutes, quadriceps, and hamstrings. It helps quantify strength capacity and guides resistance training progression safely. Proper form and supervision are critical to minimize injury risk during maximal testing.

Q100. Answer: A

Explanation: The Rockport Walk Test is ideal for deconditioned clients because it uses submaximal effort to estimate VO_2 max. It measures time to walk one mile and post-exercise heart rate, providing an accessible yet reliable assessment of cardiovascular endurance without overexertion.

Questions (101-200)

Q101. A client's blood pressure reads 142/92 mmHg. What does this indicate?

A. Normal blood pressure

B. Prehypertension

C. Hypertension (Stage 1)

D. Low blood pressure

Q102. Which postural distortion pattern involves anterior pelvic tilt and increased lumbar lordosis?

A. Upper crossed syndrome

B. Lower crossed syndrome

C. Pronation distortion syndrome

D. Posterior pelvic tilt syndrome

Q103. During a single-leg squat assessment, the client's knee moves inward. Which muscle is likely underactive?

A. Gluteus medius

B. Tensor fasciae latae

C. Adductor longus

D. Vastus lateralis

Q104. What should a personal trainer do if a client reports dizziness during testing?

A. Continue the assessment slowly

B. Have the client sit or lie down immediately

C. Give them water and resume testing

D. Ignore it unless fainting occurs

Q105. Which movement assessment evaluates the client's ability to stabilize during upper-body pulling actions?

A. Pulling assessment

B. Push-up test

C. Bench press 1RM

D. Overhead squat

Q106. What is the purpose of a subjective lifestyle questionnaire?

A. Determine 1RM strength

B. Identify psychological and behavioral patterns

C. Measure resting heart rate

D. Assess flexibility

Q107. Which postural deviation is commonly seen in individuals with tight hip flexors?

A. Posterior pelvic tilt

B. Flat lumbar curve

C. Neutral spine

D. Anterior pelvic tilt

Q108. Which movement assessment is most useful for identifying shoulder and core stability during dynamic motion?

A. Single-leg squat

B. Push-up with rotation

C. Overhead squat

D. Pulling assessment

Q109. Which of the following represents a proper sequence of assessments?

A. Movement → Subjective → Objective

B. Objective → Movement → Cardiorespiratory

C. Subjective → Objective → Movement
D. Flexibility → Postural → Subjective

Q110. Which of the following assessments directly measures muscular endurance?
A. Bench press 1RM
B. Push-up test
C. Vertical jump test
D. Overhead squat

Q111. What does a heart rate recovery assessment measure?
A. Cardiovascular efficiency
B. Muscular power output
C. Resting metabolic rate
D. Lung capacity

Q112. Which client would benefit most from postural assessment before performance testing?
A. Competitive athlete
B. Deconditioned office worker
C. Endurance runner
D. Experienced lifter

Q113. What is the purpose of circumference measurements?
A. Estimate body composition and track fat loss
B. Measure cardiorespiratory endurance
C. Evaluate postural alignment
D. Assess muscular strength

Q114. Which muscle imbalance is indicated by knees caving inward during an overhead squat?
A. Overactive gluteus medius
B. Underactive adductors
C. Underactive gluteus medius
D. Overactive biceps femoris

Q115. What should a trainer do if a client reports taking beta-blocker medication?
A. Avoid cardiorespiratory training
B. Use RPE instead of heart rate to gauge intensity
C. Increase target heart rate zones
D. Focus only on resistance training

Q116. What is the primary purpose of performing a movement assessment before designing a workout program?
A. To identify fitness goals
B. To evaluate compensations and movement inefficiencies
C. To measure cardiovascular capacity
D. To estimate resting metabolism

Q117. Which test estimates a client's aerobic capacity without requiring maximal exertion?
A. 1.5-Mile Run
B. Cooper 12-Minute Run
C. Rockport Walk Test
D. Bruce Treadmill Test

Q118. A client's head protrudes forward during a postural assessment. Which muscle is most likely overactive?
A. Deep cervical flexors
B. Upper trapezius
C. Levator scapulae

D. Sternocleidomastoid

Q119. During the overhead squat, the client's arms fall forward. Which muscle is underactive?

A. Latissimus dorsi

B. Teres major

C. Mid/lower trapezius

D. Pectoralis minor

Q120. Which physiological variable decreases as a result of improved cardiorespiratory fitness?

A. Resting heart rate

B. Stroke volume

C. VO_2 max

D. Cardiac output

Q121. What is the main purpose of a postural assessment?

A. To test muscular endurance

B. To identify deviations from ideal alignment

C. To evaluate energy system efficiency

D. To determine heart rate zones

Q122. What does an elevated heart rate during light exercise suggest?

A. Efficient aerobic metabolism

B. Fatigue or dehydration

C. Improved cardiac output

D. Low cardiovascular stress

Q123. A client's feet turn outward during the overhead squat. Which muscles are overactive?

A. Gastrocnemius and biceps femoris

B. Gluteus medius and minimus

C. Vastus medialis oblique and adductors

D. Hamstrings and tibialis anterior

Q124. What information does the talk test provide?

A. Resting heart rate

B. Anaerobic threshold estimation

C. Flexibility level

D. VO_2 max prediction

Q125. Which movement pattern is assessed in the single-leg squat test?

A. Hip extension

B. Trunk rotation

C. Shoulder abduction

D. Frontal plane stability and knee alignment

Q126. A client with rounded shoulders and a forward head posture likely has which underactive muscles?

A. Pectoralis major and levator scapulae

B. Rhomboids and deep cervical flexors

C. Latissimus dorsi and teres major

D. Upper trapezius and sternocleidomastoid

Q127. Which assessment identifies potential muscle imbalances within the lumbo-pelvic-hip complex?

A. Push-up test

B. Overhead squat test

C. Rockport walk test

D. Step-up test

Q128. What is the proper order of conducting assessments during an initial session?

A. Subjective → Objective → Movement → Performance
B. Objective → Performance → Subjective → Movement
C. Movement → Objective → Subjective → Performance
D. Performance → Movement → Objective → Subjective

Q129. Which cardiorespiratory test is most suitable for a sedentary individual?
A. Cooper 12-Minute Run
B. 1.5-Mile Run
C. Step test
D. VO_2 max treadmill test

Q130. Which test evaluates muscular strength of the upper body?
A. Bench press 1RM test
B. Rockport Walk Test
C. Push-up endurance test
D. Pulling assessment

Q131. A client demonstrates excessive arching of the lower back during the overhead squat. Which muscle is likely overactive?
A. Gluteus maximus
B. Hip flexors
C. Hamstrings
D. External obliques

Q132. Which assessment measures dynamic flexibility, core strength, and balance together?
A. Overhead squat test
B. Step-up test
C. Rockport walk test
D. Push-up test

Q133. What is the recommended rest period between repeated assessments to ensure accuracy?
A. 15 seconds
B. 30 seconds
C. 1–2 minutes
D. 5–10 minutes

Q134. A client's blood pressure is recorded as 128/84 mmHg. How should this be classified?
A. Normal
B. Elevated
C. Stage 1 hypertension
D. Stage 2 hypertension

Q135. Which factor can affect accuracy of skinfold body composition testing?
A. Environmental temperature
B. Resting heart rate
C. Training experience
D. Sleep duration

Q136. During a pulling assessment, the client's shoulders elevate. Which muscles are overactive?
A. Lower trapezius
B. Upper trapezius and levator scapulae
C. Rhomboids
D. Serratus anterior

Q137. Which test assesses lower-body power output?
A. Vertical jump test
B. Step test

C. Rockport walk test
D. Push-up test

Q138. Which of the following assessments would best determine a client's movement efficiency under load?

A. Overhead squat
B. Deadlift pattern test
C. Step-up test
D. 1.5-Mile Run

Q139. Which physiological measurement is most indicative of aerobic endurance capacity?

A. Resting heart rate
B. Blood pressure
C. VO_2 max
D. Lactate threshold

Q140. Which factor can alter heart rate response during assessments?

A. Hydration status and temperature
B. Hair length
C. Clothing color
D. Time of year

Q141. What is the primary goal of the fitness assessment process?

A. To sell more training sessions
B. To establish a safe and effective starting point
C. To test the client's pain threshold
D. To compare clients against athletic standards

Q142. Which assessment evaluates dynamic flexibility, core control, and balance simultaneously?

A. Rockport walk test
B. Single-leg squat assessment
C. Overhead squat assessment
D. Step test

Q143. A client reports knee pain during squatting movements. What should the trainer do first?

A. Immediately increase knee flexion range
B. Refer to a medical professional for clearance
C. Provide heavier resistance
D. Ignore discomfort and continue

Q144. Which test is most appropriate for measuring static balance?

A. Single-leg balance test
B. Step-up test
C. Vertical jump test
D. Push-up test

Q145. What type of assessment provides measurable physiological data?

A. Subjective assessment
B. Behavioral assessment
C. Psychological assessment
D. Objective assessment

Q146. Which test determines maximal oxygen consumption?

A. Rockport Walk Test
B. YMCA Step Test
C. VO_2 Max Test
D. 1-Repetition Maximum

Q147. What does an overactive tensor fasciae latae commonly cause during movement assessments?
A. Excessive foot pronation
B. Knee valgus (inward movement)
C. Excessive hip extension
D. Scapular elevation
Q148. What is the primary objective of a physiological assessment?
A. To evaluate range of motion
B. To measure resting and exercise responses of the cardiovascular system
C. To determine muscle fiber type distribution
D. To analyze mental focus under stress
Q149. A client's heart rate drops from 170 bpm to 120 bpm one minute post-exercise. What does this suggest?
A. Poor cardiovascular conditioning
B. Excellent recovery and aerobic fitness
C. Inaccurate measurement
D. Overtraining
Q150. What does BMI primarily estimate?
A. Bone density
B. Fat-free mass
C. Relative body weight to height
D. Hydration status
Q151. Which movement compensation is most likely with overactive adductors?
A. Knees moving outward
B. Knees caving inward
C. Feet turning inward
D. Excessive lumbar extension
Q152. What is the main benefit of conducting reassessments periodically?
A. To justify session costs
B. To evaluate progress and adjust programs accordingly
C. To maintain client entertainment
D. To promote competition between clients
Q153. Which test evaluates a client's upper-body muscular endurance?
A. Push-up test
B. Bench press 1RM
C. Vertical jump test
D. Step test
Q154. During a pulling assessment, the client exhibits low-back arching. Which muscle is likely underactive?
A. Erector spinae
B. Gluteus maximus
C. Latissimus dorsi
D. Core stabilizers
Q155. Which assessment evaluates coordination and balance on one leg while performing movement?
A. Step-up test
B. Single-leg squat assessment
C. Rockport walk test
D. Vertical jump test
Q156. What does an increased resting heart rate over several days likely indicate?

A. Overtraining or fatigue
B. Improved recovery
C. Enhanced cardiovascular function
D. Dehydration resolution

Q157. A client exhibits excessive anterior pelvic tilt during the overhead squat. Which corrective strategy is best?

A. Strengthen hip flexors and stretch glutes
B. Stretch hip flexors and strengthen glutes
C. Stretch hamstrings only
D. Focus on calf mobility only

Q158. Which assessment would best determine muscular power?

A. Push-up test
B. Bench press 1RM
C. Medicine ball chest pass
D. Rockport walk test

Q159. What should a trainer do if a client experiences shortness of breath during a step test?

A. Encourage completion
B. Stop the test immediately
C. Lower the step height
D. Wait until symptoms worsen

Q160. Which factor primarily influences postural alignment?

A. Sleep quality
B. Reaction time
C. Hydration levels
D. Muscle length and tension relationships

Q161. Which movement assessment is most useful for identifying asymmetries between limbs?

A. Rockport walk test
B. Single-leg squat assessment
C. Push-up test
D. Step test

Q162. Which type of assessment is most affected by dehydration?

A. Balance assessment
B. Flexibility assessment
C. Cardiorespiratory assessment
D. Postural assessment

Q163. What does the waist-to-hip ratio evaluate?

A. Muscular symmetry
B. Cardiovascular endurance
C. Risk for chronic disease
D. Bone mineral density

Q164. Which muscle imbalance commonly contributes to forward-head posture?

A. Underactive pectoralis major
B. Overactive sternocleidomastoid
C. Underactive upper trapezius
D. Overactive gluteus maximus

Q165. Which postural distortion is characterized by foot pronation and internal rotation of the knees?

A. Upper crossed syndrome
B. Lower crossed syndrome

C. Pronation distortion syndrome
D. Flat back syndrome

Q166. What is the first step a trainer should take before beginning any client assessments?
A. Measure resting heart rate
B. Review medical history and obtain informed consent
C. Conduct postural screening
D. Begin light warm-up activity

Q167. A client demonstrates an excessive forward lean during the overhead squat. Which corrective focus is most appropriate?
A. Strengthen calves
B. Stretch hip flexors and calves
C. Stretch glutes and hamstrings
D. Strengthen hamstrings only

Q168. Which postural deviation is commonly associated with upper-crossed syndrome?
A. Rounded shoulders and forward head
B. Flat lumbar spine and neutral shoulders
C. Excessive anterior pelvic tilt
D. Foot pronation and knee valgus

Q169. What is the correct protocol for measuring a client's waist circumference?
A. At the narrowest point of the torso
B. At the level of the navel
C. At the widest point of the hips
D. Just below the chest

Q170. Which factor can cause inaccurate heart rate readings during assessments?
A. Caffeine intake and emotional stress
B. Warm ambient temperature only
C. Muscle soreness
D. Skin hydration

Q171. A trainer notices a client's knees move outward during the overhead squat. Which muscle is likely underactive?
A. Adductors
B. Gluteus medius
C. Piriformis
D. Tensor fasciae latae

Q172. Which body composition assessment uses electrical current to estimate fat mass?
A. Hydrostatic weighing
B. Skinfold test
C. Bioelectrical impedance analysis
D. DEXA scan

Q173. Which of the following assessments should always precede physical testing for a new client?
A. Postural assessment
B. Subjective and health-risk questionnaire
C. Step test
D. Strength test

Q174. During the pushing assessment, a client's shoulders elevate. Which muscle group is overactive?
A. Upper trapezius and levator scapulae
B. Serratus anterior and rhomboids
C. Lower trapezius and rotator cuff

D. Pectoralis minor and biceps brachii

Q175. Which test would best assess an athlete's agility and quick directional change?

A. Step test

B. Pro-agility shuttle test

C. Rockport walk test

D. Push-up test

Q176. What is the main reason to reassess body composition periodically?

A. To detect hydration levels

B. To evaluate training progress and adjust goals

C. To test equipment accuracy

D. To compare against others

Q177. Which variable is assessed during the YMCA 3-Minute Step Test?

A. Resting metabolic rate

B. Muscle endurance

C. Maximal oxygen consumption

D. Recovery heart rate

Q178. What is the proper procedure when taking a radial pulse?

A. Use the thumb and apply firm pressure

B. Use index and middle fingers, apply light pressure

C. Use palm contact only

D. Measure at the elbow crease

Q179. What condition does the PAR-Q aim to identify before exercise testing?

A. Poor muscular strength

B. Cardiovascular, metabolic, or orthopedic risk factors

C. Lack of motivation

D. Poor coordination

Q180. What should a trainer do if postural assessment reveals significant asymmetry or pain?

A. Continue testing for confirmation

B. Modify the workout accordingly

C. Refer to a qualified medical professional

D. Ignore unless the client complains

Q181. When performing a squat, what is the correct kinetic chain checkpoint for knee alignment?

A. Knees tracking inward

B. Knees aligned over the second and third toes

C. Knees extending past the toes

D. Knees locked at the top

Q182. What is the optimal breathing technique during a resistance exercise like the bench press?

A. Inhale during the concentric phase

B. Hold breath throughout the set

C. Exhale during the concentric phase

D. Exhale during the eccentric phase

Q183. What is the main purpose of performing core stabilization exercises?

A. Increase maximal strength

B. Enhance neuromuscular control and trunk stability

C. Improve power production

D. Increase hypertrophy in abdominal muscles

Q184. Which flexibility technique involves holding a stretch for 30 seconds to improve range of motion?

A. Ballistic stretching

B. Static stretching
C. Active-isolated stretching
D. Dynamic stretching

Q185. During a plank exercise, which muscle acts as the primary stabilizer of the lumbar spine?
A. Transverse abdominis
B. Rectus abdominis
C. Latissimus dorsi
D. Erector spinae

Q186. Which cue is most effective for teaching proper shoulder position during a push-up?
A. Shrug shoulders up toward ears
B. Keep shoulders depressed and retracted
C. Round shoulders forward
D. Elevate chest excessively

Q187. What is the proper spotting technique during a barbell bench press?
A. Stand at the lifter's feet
B. Spot at the elbows
C. Use an alternating grip close to the bar
D. Allow the client to lift independently

Q188. When performing a lunge, which kinetic checkpoint is most important for lower-body stability?
A. Front knee behind the heel
B. Front knee aligned with the toes
C. Front knee collapsing inward
D. Torso leaning forward

Q189. Which phase of the OPT model emphasizes controlled tempo and stability before progressing to power movements?
A. Maximal Strength Training
B. Stabilization Endurance Training
C. Strength Endurance Training
D. Power Training

Q190. Which cue best assists a client struggling with excessive spinal arch during a squat?
A. "Stick your chest out"
B. "Tuck your tailbone slightly and brace your core"
C. "Lift your heels off the ground"
D. "Lean forward more"

Q191. What is the proper spotting position for a dumbbell shoulder press?
A. At the lifter's elbows
B. In front of the lifter
C. From the side, holding the bar
D. Standing behind the lifter, at the wrists

Q192. What is the purpose of performing balance training on unstable surfaces?
A. Build muscle hypertrophy
B. Enhance joint stability and proprioception
C. Increase maximal strength
D. Improve anaerobic capacity

Q193. Which flexibility technique should be avoided before power or speed activities?
A. Dynamic stretching
B. Active stretching
C. Ballistic stretching

D. Static stretching

Q194. During a push-up, the client's hips sag toward the floor. Which muscle group is likely underactive?

A. Gluteus maximus and core stabilizers

B. Quadriceps

C. Pectoralis major

D. Hip flexors

Q195. What is the ideal foot position during a standing overhead press?

A. Feet together

B. One foot slightly staggered

C. Feet wide apart

D. On toes

Q196. Which flexibility method combines active stretching and contraction of the target muscle group?

A. Static stretching

B. PNF stretching

C. Ballistic stretching

D. Dynamic stretching

Q197. During a deadlift, maintaining a neutral spine prevents which common issue?

A. Excessive glute engagement

B. Lumbar flexion and lower back strain

C. Reduced core activation

D. Overuse of quadriceps

Q198. Which cue helps improve balance during a single-leg squat?

A. Look down at the ground

B. Swing arms for balance

C. Keep eyes fixed on a point ahead

D. Shift weight to the toes

Q199. What is the primary benefit of eccentric training in resistance exercises?

A. Improves muscle relaxation

B. Enhances strength and muscle control through lengthening contractions

C. Reduces metabolic stress

D. Decreases time under tension

Q200. During a kettlebell swing, what is the primary muscle responsible for hip extension?

A. Hamstrings

B. Gluteus maximus

C. Quadriceps

D. Erector spinae

Answer keys and Explanations (101-200)

Q101. Answer: C

Explanation: A reading above 140/90 mmHg indicates Stage 1 hypertension, requiring medical clearance before high-intensity training. Trainers should avoid maximal exertion testing and focus initially on lifestyle modifications, including gradual aerobic conditioning and nutrition support within scope of practice.

Q102. Answer: B

Explanation: Lower crossed syndrome is characterized by anterior pelvic tilt and excessive lumbar arch due to tight hip flexors and weak gluteals. This imbalance affects core stability and movement efficiency. Corrective strategies include lengthening the hip flexors and strengthening the abdominals and gluteus maximus.

Q103. Answer: A

Explanation: The gluteus medius stabilizes the knee during single-leg activities. Weakness here allows femoral internal rotation and adduction, causing the knee to collapse inward. Strengthening this muscle improves hip stability and alignment during dynamic movement.

Q104. Answer: B

Explanation: Dizziness during assessment signals potential circulatory or vestibular distress. The trainer must stop testing immediately, have the client sit or lie down, and monitor vital signs. Safety is the top priority, and medical clearance should be obtained before continuing any physical testing.

Q105. Answer: A

Explanation: The pulling assessment tests upper-body pulling patterns and scapular stabilization. It identifies compensations such as shoulder elevation or trunk rotation, revealing imbalances in posterior chain muscles. This assessment helps refine programming for improved posture and back strength.

Q106. Answer: B

Explanation: Lifestyle questionnaires gather behavioral data such as stress levels, sleep habits, and nutrition. These subjective insights help trainers tailor holistic programs that support adherence, energy balance, and sustainable progress beyond physical performance measures.

Q107. Answer: D

Explanation: Tight hip flexors pull the pelvis forward, resulting in an anterior tilt and increased lumbar curvature. This distortion disrupts core alignment and can cause lower-back discomfort. Corrective focus involves stretching the hip flexors and activating the gluteus maximus and abdominals.

Q108. Answer: B

Explanation: The push-up with rotation challenges shoulder and core stabilization simultaneously. It reveals asymmetries or weaknesses in trunk control and scapular stability. This movement integrates strength and balance, making it valuable for designing corrective and functional upper-body training programs.

Q109. Answer: C

Explanation: Assessments should progress from least to most physically demanding: start with subjective data, then gather objective measures (e.g., heart rate, blood pressure), and finish with movement and performance testing. This order prioritizes safety and ensures accuracy without pre-fatiguing clients.

Q110. Answer: B

Explanation: The push-up test evaluates muscular endurance by measuring how many repetitions a client can perform with proper form. It gauges the upper-body's capacity for sustained submaximal effort and helps track progress over time through improved repetition counts.

Q111. Answer: A

Explanation: Heart rate recovery measures how quickly heart rate declines after exercise, reflecting cardiovascular efficiency and autonomic balance. Faster recovery indicates better aerobic conditioning and parasympathetic dominance, key markers of improved heart health and endurance performance.

Q112. Answer: B

Explanation: Deconditioned individuals often develop postural imbalances from sedentary behavior. Performing a postural assessment first identifies limitations or muscle imbalances that must be corrected to prevent injury when progressing to strength or endurance tests.

Q113. Answer: A

Explanation: Circumference measurements track changes in body girth at key sites such as waist, hips, arms, and thighs. These measurements estimate fat distribution and overall body composition progress, offering a practical alternative when advanced testing tools are unavailable.

Q114. Answer: C

Explanation: Weakness in the gluteus medius reduces lateral hip stability, allowing knees to move inward during squats. Strengthening this muscle improves alignment and knee tracking, reducing injury risk during lower-body training.

Q115. Answer: B

Explanation: Beta-blockers lower heart rate response to exercise, making heart rate-based intensity targets unreliable. Trainers should use the Rate of Perceived Exertion (RPE) scale to monitor effort safely while respecting medication effects on cardiovascular response.

Q116. Answer: B

Explanation: A movement assessment identifies musculoskeletal imbalances, compensations, and neuromuscular inefficiencies that may limit performance or increase injury risk. By analyzing how the body moves, trainers can pinpoint overactive and underactive muscles, then design corrective programs that enhance stability, mobility, and coordination. This step ensures safe and effective progression toward performance or aesthetic goals.

Q117. Answer: C

Explanation: The Rockport Walk Test uses submaximal effort to estimate VO_2 max by having a client walk one mile as fast as possible. Post-exercise heart rate and completion time determine aerobic capacity. It's ideal for beginners, older adults, and deconditioned clients, minimizing risk while providing valuable data for cardiovascular training recommendations.

Q118. Answer: D

Explanation: The sternocleidomastoid becomes overactive in forward-head posture, pulling the head anteriorly and placing stress on cervical structures. This imbalance often accompanies underactive deep cervical flexors. Corrective programming should focus on stretching the sternocleidomastoid and strengthening deep neck stabilizers to restore alignment and reduce neck strain.

Q119. Answer: C

Explanation: Weakness in the mid and lower trapezius contributes to the arms falling forward by reducing scapular retraction and upward rotation. Strengthening these muscles enhances shoulder stability and alignment during dynamic overhead movements, improving posture and reducing stress on the upper back and shoulders.

Q120. Answer: A

Explanation: As cardiovascular efficiency improves, resting heart rate decreases because the heart becomes stronger and pumps more blood per beat. This adaptation reduces workload on the heart while maintaining oxygen delivery. A lower resting heart rate reflects enhanced aerobic conditioning and recovery capacity.

Q121. Answer: B

Explanation: Postural assessment identifies deviations from ideal skeletal alignment caused by muscle imbalances, habitual positions, or injury. Recognizing these deviations allows trainers to design corrective exercises that restore joint positioning, improve movement mechanics, and prevent overuse injuries during training and daily life.

Q122. Answer: B

Explanation: An abnormally high heart rate during light effort may signal dehydration, fatigue, or insufficient recovery. The heart compensates by increasing rate to maintain oxygen delivery. Monitoring this response helps trainers detect early signs of overtraining or stress, prompting rest or hydration adjustments.

Q123. Answer: A

Explanation: Tightness in the gastrocnemius and biceps femoris externally rotates the feet, creating compensation during squats. This pattern limits proper alignment and can increase stress on the knees. Corrective strategies include stretching these muscles and strengthening the adductors and medial hamstrings for improved alignment.

Q124. Answer: B

Explanation: The talk test estimates anaerobic threshold by evaluating the point at which speaking becomes difficult during exercise. As intensity increases and ventilation rises, the body transitions from aerobic to anaerobic metabolism. This simple, practical method helps trainers gauge intensity levels for effective cardiovascular training without advanced equipment.

Q125. Answer: D

Explanation: The single-leg squat test evaluates frontal plane stability and knee alignment by observing dynamic control of the hip, knee, and ankle. It highlights weaknesses in the gluteus medius and core stabilizers that can lead to faulty mechanics and injury risk during unilateral movements.

Q126. Answer: B

Explanation: Rounded shoulders and forward head posture often involve underactive rhomboids and deep cervical flexors. These muscles maintain scapular retraction and cervical alignment. Strengthening them corrects upper-crossed posture, reduces neck strain, and improves shoulder mechanics during pressing and pulling exercises.

Q127. Answer: B

Explanation: The overhead squat test reveals movement dysfunctions within the lumbo-pelvic-hip complex, such as excessive arching or anterior pelvic tilt. By observing compensations, trainers can pinpoint overactive hip flexors and underactive glutes or core stabilizers, informing corrective programming that restores optimal kinetic-chain function.

Q128. Answer: A

Explanation: Assessments should progress from least to most demanding: gather subjective data first (health history), then objective data (vitals and measurements), followed by movement and performance testing. This systematic flow ensures safety, efficiency, and accurate interpretation of results without prematurely fatiguing the client.

Q129. Answer: C

Explanation: The step test provides a submaximal measure of cardiorespiratory endurance suitable for sedentary or deconditioned clients. It involves stepping up and down for a fixed duration and evaluating recovery heart rate. This low-impact assessment safely gauges aerobic fitness without excessive cardiovascular strain.

Q130. Answer: A

Explanation: The bench press 1RM test determines maximal upper-body strength by identifying the greatest weight a client can lift once with proper form. This test quantifies strength levels and informs load progression while maintaining controlled, supervised conditions for safety.

Q131. Answer: B

Explanation: Overactive hip flexors, particularly the iliopsoas, pull the pelvis anteriorly, producing excessive lumbar arching during squats. This imbalance stresses the lower back and decreases core stability. Corrective training includes stretching the hip flexors and activating gluteal and core muscles.

Q132. Answer: A

Explanation: The overhead squat test simultaneously challenges flexibility, core strength, and neuromuscular balance. Observing movement quality across planes reveals compensations and imbalances affecting performance. Its integrated nature makes it a cornerstone of NASM's kinetic chain assessment strategy.

Q133. Answer: C

Explanation: Allowing 1–2 minutes between repeated assessment trials helps restore cardiovascular stability and ensures consistent effort across tests. This rest period prevents fatigue from skewing results, maintaining accuracy and reliability in data collection.

Q134. Answer: B

Explanation: A reading of 120–129 systolic and below 80 diastolic is considered elevated, indicating early risk of hypertension. While not yet hypertensive, the client should monitor lifestyle factors and avoid excessive cardiovascular strain until blood pressure normalizes through conditioning and nutrition.

Q135. Answer: A

Explanation: Skinfold accuracy can be influenced by environmental temperature, as warm conditions increase skin elasticity and hydration. Proper calibration, consistent site selection, and technician skill are critical for reliable measurements, making environmental control an important part of standardized testing.

Q136. Answer: B

Explanation: Overactivity in the upper trapezius and levator scapulae elevates the shoulders during pulling motions. This imbalance disrupts scapular stability and reduces pulling efficiency. Stretching these muscles and strengthening the lower trapezius and serratus anterior improves posture and shoulder mechanics.

Q137. Answer: A

Explanation: The vertical jump test measures explosive lower-body power by evaluating jump height from a static position. It reflects neuromuscular efficiency and fast-twitch fiber recruitment, essential for athletic performance. Tracking improvements indicates enhanced power development from plyometric or strength training.

Q138. Answer: B

Explanation: The deadlift pattern test evaluates integrated movement efficiency, spinal alignment, and hip mechanics under load. It reveals compensation patterns during complex lifting tasks, providing insight into real-world performance and risk of lower-back strain.

Q139. Answer: C

Explanation: VO_2 max represents the maximum volume of oxygen the body can utilize during intense exercise, serving as the gold standard for aerobic endurance. Higher VO_2 max values correlate with improved cardiovascular efficiency, oxygen transport, and stamina across prolonged physical activity.

Q140. Answer: A

Explanation: Dehydration, caffeine intake, emotional stress, and ambient temperature can elevate heart rate readings, reducing accuracy in fitness assessments. Controlling these factors ensures reliable measurement of true cardiovascular performance and exercise readiness.

Q141. Answer: B

Explanation: The assessment process establishes a baseline of a client's health, posture, and movement capacity, allowing for the safe design of personalized programs. By identifying strengths, limitations, and potential risks, trainers can structure progressive exercise plans that enhance performance, reduce injury risk, and align with the client's fitness goals.

Q142. Answer: C
Explanation: The overhead squat assessment evaluates multiple components—dynamic flexibility, core control, balance, and neuromuscular efficiency—through coordinated multi-joint motion. Observing compensations provides insights into overactive and underactive muscles. This integrated test allows trainers to design corrective strategies that enhance movement quality and performance.
Q143. Answer: B
Explanation: Any report of joint pain, especially knee discomfort, requires referral to a licensed medical professional before continuing assessment or exercise. Trainers must operate within scope of practice and prioritize client safety, ensuring no structural damage is exacerbated during testing or training.
Q144. Answer: A
Explanation: The single-leg balance test isolates static postural control by assessing a client's ability to maintain equilibrium on one leg without movement. It highlights deficits in proprioception and stabilization, providing valuable feedback for improving neuromuscular coordination and lower-extremity stability.
Q145. Answer: D
Explanation: Objective assessments collect measurable data such as heart rate, blood pressure, circumference, or performance metrics. These quantifiable outcomes track progress and training effectiveness. They complement subjective information to provide a comprehensive understanding of a client's health and fitness status.
Q146. Answer: C
Explanation: A VO_2 Max Test directly measures the body's capacity to utilize oxygen during incremental exercise to exhaustion. It represents aerobic endurance potential and overall cardiovascular efficiency. Although equipment-intensive, it provides the most precise measure of aerobic performance capability.
Q147. Answer: B
Explanation: The tensor fasciae latae, when overactive, contributes to knee valgus by internally rotating and adducting the femur. This compensation disrupts alignment during squats or lunges. Stretching the TFL and strengthening the gluteus medius restore balance and proper knee tracking.
Q148. Answer: B
Explanation: Physiological assessments gauge cardiovascular efficiency through metrics like resting heart rate, blood pressure, and recovery heart rate. These parameters reflect heart health and aerobic conditioning, allowing trainers to set intensity zones and monitor adaptation over time.
Q149. Answer: B
Explanation: A rapid decrease in heart rate during the first minute of recovery indicates strong parasympathetic response and cardiovascular efficiency. Faster recovery times reflect improved oxygen delivery, metabolic waste clearance, and aerobic fitness, confirming effective endurance conditioning.
Q150. Answer: C
Explanation: Body Mass Index (BMI) is a ratio of weight to height used to categorize individuals into weight classifications. Though it doesn't distinguish between muscle and fat, BMI helps identify general health risks associated with obesity or underweight status, guiding further assessment.
Q151. Answer: B
Explanation: Overactive adductors pull the knees toward the midline, creating valgus movement during squats. This faulty alignment stresses knee structures and disrupts hip stability. Stretching the adductors and strengthening the gluteus medius help restore balance and correct the pattern.
Q152. Answer: B
Explanation: Periodic reassessments track progress, evaluate training effectiveness, and guide necessary program adjustments. Objective improvements in posture, strength, or endurance confirm adaptations and motivate clients, while stagnation signals the need for modifications to maintain progress.
Q153. Answer: A

Explanation: The push-up test measures upper-body endurance by counting the number of properly executed repetitions before fatigue. This provides a practical indicator of the muscular stamina required for sustained submaximal efforts during daily and athletic activities.

Q154. Answer: D

Explanation: Weak core stabilizers allow excessive lumbar extension during pulling exercises. Strengthening the transverse abdominis and internal obliques improves spinal stability and alignment, reducing stress on the lower back and promoting efficient kinetic-chain movement during resistance training.

Q155. Answer: B

Explanation: The single-leg squat assessment challenges coordination, balance, and strength on one leg. Observing deviations provides insight into hip and core stability deficits. It's a valuable screening tool for detecting lower-extremity imbalances affecting dynamic control and athletic movement.

Q156. Answer: A

Explanation: A rising resting heart rate over consecutive days often signals fatigue or overtraining. It reflects autonomic nervous system stress and insufficient recovery. Monitoring this trend allows trainers to adjust workloads, prevent burnout, and support sustainable adaptation through adequate rest.

Q157. Answer: B

Explanation: Excessive anterior pelvic tilt results from tight hip flexors and weak glutes. Corrective action includes stretching the hip flexors and reinforcing gluteal activation to restore pelvic neutrality. Balancing these opposing muscle groups improves posture and movement quality during squats and daily activities.

Q158. Answer: C

Explanation: The medicine ball chest pass measures upper-body power by assessing explosive force production. It evaluates fast-twitch fiber engagement and neuromuscular coordination, providing insight into dynamic strength and performance potential in sport or functional tasks.

Q159. Answer: B

Explanation: Shortness of breath indicates possible cardiovascular or respiratory distress, requiring immediate cessation of activity. Safety is paramount—testing should stop, and the client should rest until symptoms resolve. Medical evaluation may be necessary before resuming assessments or training.

Q160. Answer: D

Explanation: Postural alignment depends on the balance between muscle length and tension. Overactive or shortened muscles pull joints out of alignment, while underactive muscles fail to stabilize them. Restoring optimal length-tension relationships improves symmetry, efficiency, and joint health.

Q161. Answer: B

Explanation: The single-leg squat assessment exposes side-to-side discrepancies in balance, strength, and coordination. It highlights unilateral weaknesses that may not appear during bilateral exercises. Correcting these asymmetries enhances performance and reduces the likelihood of overuse injuries.

Q162. Answer: C

Explanation: Dehydration impairs cardiovascular efficiency, raising heart rate and reducing blood volume. This directly impacts cardiorespiratory assessments by altering test results and perceived exertion. Ensuring proper hydration before testing maintains accuracy and safety during exercise evaluation.

Q163. Answer: C

Explanation: The waist-to-hip ratio compares abdominal to hip circumference, providing an indicator of visceral fat distribution. Higher ratios correlate with increased risk of cardiovascular disease, diabetes, and metabolic disorders. Monitoring this measure helps guide health and lifestyle recommendations.

Q164. Answer: B

Explanation: Overactivity in the sternocleidomastoid pulls the head forward, disrupting neutral spinal alignment. This compensation increases strain on the cervical spine and shoulders. Stretching the sternocleidomastoid while strengthening deep cervical flexors restores posture and reduces tension-related discomfort.

Q165. Answer: C

Explanation: Pronation distortion syndrome features excessive foot pronation and knee internal rotation caused by overactive peroneals and adductors and underactive gluteals. It alters kinetic chain alignment, reducing movement efficiency and predisposing the body to injuries. Corrective training focuses on strengthening the gluteus medius and improving foot stability.

Q166. Answer: B

Explanation: Reviewing medical history and obtaining informed consent ensures the client is cleared for participation and understands all assessment procedures. This step protects both client and trainer legally and ethically while identifying potential health risks that may alter or limit testing protocols.

Q167. Answer: B

Explanation: Tight hip flexors and calves contribute to forward lean by restricting hip extension and ankle dorsiflexion. Stretching these muscles restores proper movement mechanics and postural balance during squats, preventing compensatory stress on the lower back and knees.

Q168. Answer: A

Explanation: Upper-crossed syndrome involves tight pectoral and neck muscles with weak mid-back and deep neck flexors, resulting in rounded shoulders and forward head posture. Corrective programming includes stretching overactive muscles and strengthening the posterior chain for balanced alignment.

Q169. Answer: B

Explanation: Waist circumference is measured horizontally at the level of the navel, ensuring consistent placement for tracking body composition. This location reflects visceral fat distribution and correlates with risk for metabolic and cardiovascular disease, making accuracy critical for health assessment.

Q170. Answer: A

Explanation: Caffeine, anxiety, or emotional stress stimulate sympathetic nervous activity, artificially elevating heart rate readings. These variables compromise accuracy when estimating aerobic fitness or target heart rate zones, emphasizing the importance of controlling pre-test conditions.

Q171. Answer: A

Explanation: Underactive adductors fail to maintain proper knee alignment during squatting movements, allowing the knees to move outward. Strengthening these muscles restores balance between the adductors and abductors, enhancing lower-limb alignment and movement efficiency.

Q172. Answer: C

Explanation: Bioelectrical impedance analysis estimates body fat percentage by passing a harmless electrical current through the body. Because fat tissue conducts electricity poorly compared to lean mass, resistance levels reveal composition. It's quick, noninvasive, and useful for monitoring body changes over time.

Q173. Answer: B

Explanation: Completing subjective health-risk and lifestyle questionnaires before testing identifies contraindications and ensures safety. This process includes PAR-Q and medical clearance where necessary. It guides the trainer in modifying or delaying certain tests based on risk factors.

Q174. Answer: A

Explanation: Shoulder elevation during pushing indicates overactivity in the upper trapezius and levator scapulae. These muscles overpower stabilizers, disrupting scapular mechanics. Stretching them while strengthening lower trapezius and serratus anterior improves shoulder function and posture.

Q175. Answer: B

Explanation: The pro-agility shuttle test measures the ability to accelerate, decelerate, and change direction quickly. It assesses coordination, balance, and neuromuscular control—key components of agility. This makes it ideal for athletes and performance-focused clients.

Q176. Answer: B
Explanation: Regular body composition reassessments track changes in fat and lean mass, offering clear evidence of training progress. This information helps adjust exercise intensity, nutrition strategies, and motivational feedback, ensuring continuous improvement toward specific client goals.
Q177. Answer: D
Explanation: The YMCA Step Test measures recovery heart rate immediately after exercise to estimate aerobic fitness. Faster heart rate recovery indicates improved cardiovascular efficiency and conditioning, making it a simple yet effective assessment for most clients.
Q178. Answer: B
Explanation: The radial pulse is taken by placing the index and middle fingers lightly along the thumb side of the wrist. Gentle pressure prevents artery occlusion and ensures accurate detection of pulse beats for heart rate measurement.
Q179. Answer: B
Explanation: The PAR-Q screens for cardiovascular, metabolic, and orthopedic conditions that could pose health risks during exercise. Identifying these factors allows trainers to refer clients for medical clearance, ensuring assessments and programs are conducted safely.
Q180. Answer: C
Explanation: Significant asymmetry or pain observed during postural assessment suggests possible structural or neurological issues that require medical evaluation. Referring the client to a licensed healthcare provider ensures safety and maintains ethical practice boundaries within the trainer's professional scope.
Q181. Answer: B
Explanation: Proper squat form requires knees to remain aligned with the second and third toes throughout movement. This ensures balanced force distribution across the knee joint and reduces stress on ligaments. Maintaining this alignment enhances stability, prevents valgus collapse, and optimizes kinetic chain efficiency during lower-body exercises.
Q182. Answer: C
Explanation: Exhaling during the concentric phase stabilizes the core and aids force production by maintaining intra-abdominal pressure. Controlled breathing improves oxygen delivery, reduces dizziness, and enhances lifting efficiency. Proper breathing technique also minimizes blood pressure spikes and supports consistent muscular performance during multi-joint lifts.
Q183. Answer: B
Explanation: Core stabilization exercises focus on improving deep trunk muscle activation and neuromuscular control. By strengthening muscles like the transverse abdominis and multifidus, they provide spinal support, enhance balance, and create a foundation for efficient force transfer during dynamic movement and heavy lifting.
Q184. Answer: B
Explanation: Static stretching involves holding a muscle in a lengthened position for about 30 seconds, allowing the muscle spindle to relax and elongate safely. This method effectively increases joint range of motion, decreases muscle stiffness, and reduces the risk of strain during subsequent activity.
Q185. Answer: A
Explanation: The transverse abdominis serves as the body's natural weight belt by stabilizing the lumbar spine during isometric core activities like planks. It increases intra-abdominal pressure and provides deep stabilization, enhancing posture and reducing the likelihood of lower back strain.
Q186. Answer: B
Explanation: Cueing clients to keep the shoulders depressed and retracted encourages engagement of the scapular stabilizers, promoting proper upper-body alignment. This position prevents shoulder impingement, enhances core control, and allows efficient transfer of force through the kinetic chain.

Q187. Answer: C

Explanation: The correct bench press spot involves using an alternating grip close to the bar, ready to assist as needed without taking over the lift. This ensures safety while maintaining the client's control. Proper spotting prevents bar drops and ensures safe load handling throughout the set.

Q188. Answer: B

Explanation: The front knee should track directly over the toes, maintaining alignment between the hip, knee, and ankle. This prevents excessive torque at the knee joint and enhances balance, ensuring proper muscle engagement of the quadriceps and gluteals.

Q189. Answer: B

Explanation: The Stabilization Endurance phase emphasizes controlled movement, postural alignment, and neuromuscular coordination. It builds foundational control and joint integrity before advancing to higher intensity or power phases. This focus reduces injury risk while developing consistent movement efficiency.

Q190. Answer: B

Explanation: Cueing the client to tuck the tailbone slightly and brace the core encourages neutral spine alignment and pelvic stability. This correction reduces lumbar hyperextension, activates deep core stabilizers, and maintains proper posture throughout the squat movement.

Q191. Answer: D

Explanation: For the dumbbell shoulder press, spotters should stand behind the client and guide at the wrists. This placement allows immediate control if the lifter loses balance while respecting their natural pressing path. It ensures safety and reinforces stability without interfering with form.

Q192. Answer: B

Explanation: Training on unstable surfaces challenges proprioception and joint stability by requiring continuous neuromuscular adjustments. It enhances balance, coordination, and joint integrity, which translates into improved control during athletic or daily movements, especially under dynamic conditions.

Q193. Answer: D

Explanation: Static stretching temporarily reduces neural activation and force output, which can impair performance in explosive or speed-based activities. Dynamic and active stretching are preferred pre-performance to enhance range of motion while maintaining neuromuscular readiness.

Q194. Answer: A

Explanation: Sagging hips during a push-up indicate weak gluteus maximus and core stabilizers, leading to poor spinal alignment. Strengthening these muscles promotes proper lumbopelvic stability and posture during upper-body exercises, improving form and safety.

Q195. Answer: B

Explanation: A staggered stance enhances balance and reduces lumbar strain by improving base support. It stabilizes the kinetic chain and minimizes compensations from the lower back or hips during pressing movements, ensuring safe and efficient force transfer.

Q196. Answer: B

Explanation: Proprioceptive Neuromuscular Facilitation (PNF) involves alternating muscle contraction and relaxation phases to enhance flexibility. The contract-relax technique utilizes the Golgi tendon organ response, improving muscle extensibility and joint range of motion effectively.

Q197. Answer: B

Explanation: Maintaining a neutral spine during deadlifts prevents lumbar flexion and associated strain on spinal discs. Neutral alignment allows force to transfer efficiently through the posterior chain, enhancing performance while protecting the lower back from overuse injuries.

Q198. Answer: C

Explanation: Focusing the gaze forward on a fixed point improves postural control and proprioception during single-leg balance tasks. This visual stabilization enhances neuromuscular coordination and reduces wobbling, supporting overall lower-body stability.

Q199. Answer: B

Explanation: Eccentric contractions lengthen the muscle under tension, enhancing strength, control, and tissue resilience. They create high mechanical stress, promoting adaptation and joint stability while minimizing energy expenditure compared to concentric actions.

Q200. Answer: B

Explanation: The gluteus maximus drives hip extension during a kettlebell swing, generating explosive power. Proper glute activation ensures efficient posterior chain engagement and protects the lower back from compensatory strain, optimizing both power output and movement safety.

Questions (201-300)

Q201. Which variable should be monitored most closely during plyometric exercises?

A. Load
B. Rate of force production and landing mechanics
C. Duration of rest between sets
D. Breathing pattern

Q202. Which muscle primarily stabilizes the scapula during overhead pressing movements?

A. Serratus anterior
B. Trapezius (upper fibers)
C. Deltoid
D. Rhomboids

Q203. Which flexibility technique is best used post-workout to aid recovery?

A. Ballistic stretching
B. Static stretching
C. Active stretching
D. Dynamic stretching

Q204. During a standing cable row, which cue ensures proper shoulder engagement?

A. Pull with the arms only
B. Keep spine rounded
C. Shrug shoulders up during the pull
D. Lead with the elbows and squeeze the shoulder blades

Q205. What is the optimal instruction for maintaining spinal alignment during a plank?

A. Drop hips to increase challenge
B. Keep a straight line from head to heels
C. Raise hips above shoulders
D. Round the upper back

Q206. Which exercise primarily strengthens the local stabilization system of the core?

A. Back squat
B. Plank
C. Sit-up
D. Barbell row

Q207. During a lat pulldown, what is the correct movement of the scapula during the concentric phase?

A. Protraction and elevation
B Protraction and upward rotation
C.. Retraction and depression
D. Elevation and rotation

Q208. What is the most appropriate cue for a client performing a lunge with excessive forward lean?

A. "Lean forward to keep balance."
B. "Keep your chest up and engage your core."
C. "Step shorter to make it easier."
D. "Push from your toes only."

Q209. Which flexibility exercise improves hip flexor extensibility?

A. Standing quad stretch
B. Kneeling hip flexor stretch
C. Seated hamstring stretch
D. Butterfly stretch

Q210. During resistance training, why is tempo important?

A. It determines rest period length
B. It prevents muscle fatigue
C. It improves grip strength
D. It controls time under tension and movement quality

Q211. Which muscle acts as the primary mover during a seated row exercise?
A. Pectoralis major
B. Latissimus dorsi
C. Anterior deltoid
D. Rectus abdominis

Q212. What is the purpose of performing a dynamic warm-up before resistance training?
A. Reduce joint range of motion
B. Decrease body temperature
C. Activate neuromuscular pathways and increase blood flow
D. Fatigue muscles prior to lifting

Q213. Which exercise best develops balance in the sagittal plane?
A. Lateral shuffle
B. Single-leg balance reach forward
C. Side plank
D. Cable rotation

Q214. What is the primary goal of plyometric training?
A. Increase flexibility
B. Improve maximal strength
C. Enhance rate of force production
D. Build muscular endurance

Q215. Which exercise variation would regress a standard push-up?
A. Push-up on toes
B. Stability ball push-up
C. Push-up on knees
D. Decline push-up

Q216. When teaching resistance training, what type of cueing is most effective for beginners?
A. Internal-only focus
B. External and kinesthetic cues
C. Visual-only cues
D. Complex technical language

Q217. Which exercise primarily develops stabilization endurance of the core?
A. Cable rotation
B. Stability ball bridge
C. Sit-up
D. Back extension

Q218. When cueing proper breathing during a deadlift, what instruction should a trainer give?
A. "Exhale as you lift, inhale as you lower."
B. "Hold your breath the entire time."
C. "Breathe rapidly throughout."
D. "Exhale during the eccentric phase."

Q219. What is the best cue for maintaining balance during a single-leg squat?
A. "Keep weight on your toes."
B. "Drive your knee inward."
C. "Keep your chest up and your core tight."

D. “Look down at your feet.”

Q220. What is the primary function of the rotator cuff during resistance exercises?

A. Produce maximal shoulder power

B. Stabilize the glenohumeral joint

C. Move the scapula

D. Assist in wrist control

Q221. Which type of exercise would improve proprioception most effectively?

A. Machine leg press

B. Single-leg balance reach

C. Seated chest press

D. Leg curl machine

Q222. When performing the cable rotation exercise, what is the main goal?

A. Isolate arm movement

B. Focus on shoulder hypertrophy

C. Stretch the lower back

D. Enhance transverse plane core stability and rotational control

Q223. What is the safest way to spot during a back squat?

A. Stand in front of the lifter

B. Stand behind the lifter with arms near rib cage

C. Hold the barbell ends directly

D. Allow the lifter to re-rack alone

Q224. Which type of stretching involves controlled movement through a full range of motion?

A. Static stretching

B. Dynamic stretching

C. PNF stretching

D. Ballistic stretching

Q225. During a step-up exercise, which muscle is the primary mover?

A. Hamstrings

B. Quadriceps

C. Gluteus maximus

D. Soleus

Q226. Which variable is most important to control during balance training?

A. Visual input

B. Tempo and movement speed

C. External load

D. Number of repetitions

Q227. Which exercise is best suited for developing core power?

A. Medicine ball rotation throw

B. Cable chop

C. Stability ball plank

D. Side bridge

Q228. What is the primary cue for maintaining alignment in a front plank?

A. “Lift hips high to increase challenge.”

B. “Draw your navel in and keep hips level.”

C. “Relax your core and hold your breath.”

D. “Arch your back for tension.”

Q229. Which movement pattern is emphasized in kettlebell swing training?

A. Squat

B. Hip hinge
C. Lunge
D. Step-up

Q230. What is the benefit of training on a stability ball compared to the floor?
A. Increased joint stability and core activation
B. Greater muscle hypertrophy
C. Decreased range of motion
D. Improved maximal strength

Q231. During a front squat, what is the ideal bar placement?
A. On the upper trapezius
B. Across the mid-back
C. Resting on the front deltoids and clavicles
D. On the neck

Q232. What should a trainer cue to correct a client whose heels lift during a squat?
A. "Keep your weight in your toes."
B. "Push through your heels and keep your feet flat."
C. "Lift your heels higher to go deeper."
D. "Lean forward to balance."

Q233. Which exercise best develops dynamic stabilization of the shoulder joint?
A. Bicep curl
B. Dumbbell chest press
C. Stability ball push-up
D. Triceps kickback

Q234. Which flexibility technique should be performed at the end of a workout?
A. Static stretching
B. Ballistic stretching
C. Dynamic stretching
D. Active stretching

Q235. During a bench press, what is the primary action of the pectoralis major?
A. Shoulder abduction
B. Shoulder flexion and horizontal adduction
C. Shoulder extension
D. Elbow flexion

Q236. Which core exercise emphasizes rotation in the transverse plane?
A. Back extension
B. Cable woodchop
C. Plank
D. Bridge

Q237. What is the correct spotting position during a dumbbell chest press?
A. Hold under the elbows
B. Spot from the side near shoulders
C. Stand behind the bench and grasp forearms
D. Hold at the wrists

Q238. Which muscle is primarily responsible for spinal stabilization during loaded exercises?
A. Latissimus dorsi
B. Transverse abdominis
C. Biceps femoris
D. Rectus abdominis

Q239. Which stretching method uses controlled momentum to move joints through their range of motion?
A. PNF stretching
B. Static stretching
C. Ballistic stretching
D. Dynamic stretching
Q240. Which exercise strengthens both the erector spinae and gluteus maximus simultaneously?
A. Bird-dog
B. Hip bridge
C. Prone cobra
D. Back extension
Q241. What is the safest cue for clients performing resistance exercises to protect the lower back?
A. "Lock your knees."
B. "Engage your core and maintain a neutral spine."
C. "Round your back slightly."
D. "Hold your breath for stability."
Q242. Which core exercise emphasizes anti-rotation stability?
A. Side plank
B. Crunch
C. Sit-up
D. Leg raise
Q243. Which exercise progression increases balance difficulty safely?
A. Move from bilateral to unilateral stance
B. Add heavy load before mastering form
C. Increase speed before control
D. Eliminate visual focus immediately
Q244. During an overhead press, what common error indicates tight latissimus dorsi muscles?
A. Excessive arching of the lower back
B. Knees bending excessively
C. Elbows flaring outward
D. Shoulders elevating
Q245. What is the key purpose of the eccentric phase in resistance training?
A. Maximize rest
B. Promote muscle growth and control
C. Reduce time under tension
D. Increase velocity only
Q246. Which of the following improves core stability and postural endurance?
A. Seated ab crunch
B. Leg press
C. Stability ball plank hold
D. Bicep curl
Q247. During a single-leg squat, what compensation occurs if the gluteus medius is weak?
A. Knee moves inward
B. Trunk rotates outward
C. Foot lifts off the ground
D. Ankle inverts
Q248. Which exercise primarily develops power in the lower body?
A. Squat jump

B. Static lunge
C. Step-up balance
D. Wall sit

Q249. Which resistance training technique alternates upper and lower body exercises to enhance efficiency?
A. Superset
B. Circuit training
C. Split routine
D. Pyramid loading

Q250. Which flexibility exercise improves thoracic mobility?
A. Seated forward fold
B. Cat-cow stretch
C. Child's pose
D. Standing side bend

Q251. What is the trainer's key focus during client spotting?
A. Providing constant verbal correction
B. Standing far from the client
C. Helping lift most of the weight
D. Assisting only when necessary for safety

Q252. What is the goal of reactive (plyometric) core training?
A. Maintain static posture
B. Develop explosive core stability under rapid movement
C. Improve spinal flexibility
D. Increase slow-twitch endurance

Q253. What is the most effective cue to correct shoulder elevation during pulling movements?
A. "Pull with your arms only."
B. "Draw your shoulders down and back."
C. "Shrug your shoulders up."
D. "Round your upper back."

Q254. Which exercise primarily targets ankle stability?
A. Single-leg balance reach
B. Step-up
C. Seated leg curl
D. Wall sit

Q255. Which flexibility method alternates contraction and relaxation to increase range of motion?
A. Static stretching
B. PNF stretching
C. Dynamic stretching
D. Ballistic stretching

Q256. Which cue ensures proper alignment during the Romanian deadlift?
A. "Lock your knees and pull quickly."
B. "Push your hips back and keep your spine neutral."
C. "Round your lower back slightly for stretch."
D. "Lift with your arms for control."

Q257. What is the primary benefit of using a stability ball for core training?
A. Isolates abdominal muscles only
B. Reduces neural activation
C. Increases proprioceptive challenge and core activation

D. Increases resistance load significantly

Q258. During a standing cable chest press, which joint action occurs at the shoulder during the concentric phase?

A. Shoulder flexion and horizontal adduction

B. Shoulder extension

C. Shoulder abduction

D. External rotation

Q259. Which type of exercise would best enhance dynamic postural control?

A. Machine-based chest press

B. Single-leg Romanian deadlift

C. Seated shoulder press

D. Leg curl machine

Q260. What is the key purpose of proper cueing during resistance training?

A. Increase workout volume

B. Ensure movement efficiency and safe execution

C. Reduce rest time

D. Enhance hypertrophy only

Q261. What is the primary goal of the Stabilization Endurance phase in the OPT model?

A. Increase muscle hypertrophy

B. Improve neuromuscular efficiency and joint stability

C. Maximize strength output

D. Enhance power production

Q262. How many repetitions are typically prescribed for Strength Endurance training?

A. 1–5 reps

B. 6–12 reps

C. 8–12 reps per set

D. 12–20 reps

Q263. Which acute variable determines how long the muscle is under tension?

A. Intensity

B. Tempo

C. Volume

D. Frequency

Q264. During the Power phase, which training variable is emphasized?

A. Slow tempo

B. High volume

C. Maximal velocity

D. Long rest periods

Q265. What is the correct rest interval between strength sets for maximal strength development?

A. 0–60 seconds

B. 1–2 minutes

C. 3–5 minutes

D. 5–8 minutes

Q266. Which training system alternates upper and lower body exercises with minimal rest?

A. Pyramid system

B. Circuit training

C. Superset system

D. Split routine

Q267. What type of exercise is best suited for the Power phase?

A. Slow tempo, low-load movement
B. Controlled tempo, moderate load
C. Superset of strength and power movements
D. Long-duration cardio

Q268. Which adaptation is most associated with the Hypertrophy phase?
A. Muscular size increase
B. Neural recruitment
C. Joint stability
D. Rate of force development

Q269. For a beginner client, how many days per week should resistance training be performed?
A. 1–2 days
B. 2–3 days
C. 4–6 days
D. 6–7 days

Q270. What is the primary benefit of undulating periodization?
A. Focuses on one adaptation per month
B. Avoids overload
C. Eliminates recovery periods
D. Varies intensity and volume daily or weekly

Q271. Which factor determines progression in the OPT model?
A. Training environment
B. Client's current adaptation level
C. Equipment availability
D. Session length

Q272. How many sets per exercise are typically performed during Stabilization Endurance training?
A. 1–2
B. 2–3
C. 3–4
D. 4–6

Q273. In the OPT model, which phase uses heavy loads (85–100% 1RM) for 1–5 repetitions?
A. Power
B. Strength Endurance
C. Maximal Strength
D. Hypertrophy

Q274. What type of resistance is recommended for Stabilization Endurance training?
A. Machines only
B. Free weights and body weight
C. High-load resistance
D. Variable resistance

Q275. What rest interval supports hypertrophy development?
A. 0–60 seconds
B. 2–3 minutes
C. 3–5 minutes
D. 5+ minutes

Q276. Which term describes the total amount of work performed during a session?
A. Volume
B. Frequency
C. Intensity

D. Tempo
Q277. In the Strength Endurance phase, which type of superset is performed?
A. Power with speed
B. Strength followed by stabilization
C. Hypertrophy with maximal strength
D. Balance with flexibility
Q278. What is the main goal of the Power phase in the OPT model?
A. Improve endurance
B. Enhance stabilization
C. Increase rate of force production
D. Build muscular size
Q279. Which exercise best represents a power movement?
A. Step-up
B. Medicine ball slam
C. Push-up
D. Plank
Q280. What is the primary goal of Strength Endurance training?
A. Improve joint stability
B. Develop muscular endurance and prime mover strength
C. Maximize power output
D. Increase flexibility
Q281. For a client aiming to build muscular endurance, which repetition range is optimal?
A. 1–5
B. 6–12
C. 12–20
D. 20–30
Q282. What is the recommended tempo for Stabilization Endurance training?
A. 4/2/1 (eccentric/isometric/concentric)
B. 2/0/2
C. Explosive
D. 1/1/1
Q283. How long should rest intervals be in Power training?
A. 0–30 seconds
B. 1–2 minutes
C. 3–5 minutes
D. 5–8 minutes
Q284. Which training phase typically involves 3–5 sets of 4–6 repetitions?
A. Hypertrophy
B. Strength Endurance
C. Stabilization Endurance
D. Maximal Strength
Q285. Which system is most effective for building hypertrophy?
A. Single-set
B. Superset
C. Pyramid system
D. Split routine
Q286. What is the training frequency for experienced athletes in the Power phase?
A. 1–2 sessions/week

B. 2–4 sessions/week
C. 4–6 sessions/week
D. 7 sessions/week

Q287. Which training phase uses the highest total volume?
A. Hypertrophy
B. Power
C. Stabilization Endurance
D. Maximal Strength

Q288. Which acute variable most influences the training adaptation achieved?
A. Frequency
B. Intensity
C. Order of exercises
D. Tempo

Q289. Which exercise pairing exemplifies a Power phase superset?
A. Bench press + push-up
B. Squat + jump squat
C. Bicep curl + hammer curl
D. Row + pull-up

Q290. For Strength Endurance, which rest interval is appropriate between supersets?
A. 0–60 seconds
B. 90 seconds
C. 3–5 minutes
D. 5–8 minutes

Q291. What is the best initial exercise order for total-body workouts?
A. Isolation to compound
B. Small to large muscles
C. Multi-joint to single-joint
D. Randomized sequence

Q292. In which OPT phase would tempo be fastest?
A. Stabilization
B. Hypertrophy
C. Strength Endurance
D. Power

Q293. What intensity range defines Hypertrophy training?
A. 40–60% 1RM
B. 65–75% 1RM
C. 75–85% 1RM
D. 90–100% 1RM

Q294. What repetition range defines Maximal Strength training?
A. 1–5 reps
B. 6–12 reps
C. 12–20 reps
D. 20–30 reps

Q295. Which acute variable combination defines Power training?
A. Low load, high speed
B. High volume, low rest
C. Moderate load, slow tempo
D. High load, slow tempo

Q296. What rest period supports muscular endurance?
A. 0–60 seconds
B. 90 seconds
C. 3–5 minutes
D. 5–8 minutes
Q297. Which exercise would best suit a beginner in the Stabilization phase?
A. Machine chest press
B. Stability ball push-up
C. Barbell squat
D. Power clean
Q298. Which variable primarily determines exercise intensity?
A. Rest duration
B. Load relative to 1RM
C. Training frequency
D. Exercise order
Q299. What is the goal of active rest days within a program?
A. Promote total inactivity
B. Enhance recovery through low-intensity activity
C. Increase training load
D. Reduce caloric expenditure
Q300. What is the main purpose of periodization in program design?
A. Avoid overload
B. Provide structured progression and recovery
C. Maintain constant intensity
D. Eliminate rest days

Answer keys and Explanations (201-300)

Q201. Answer: B

Explanation: In plyometric training, monitoring the rate of force production and proper landing mechanics ensures safety and performance. Controlled landings with soft knees and neutral alignment protect joints, while efficient force output enhances explosive capability and coordination.

Q202. Answer: A

Explanation: The serratus anterior maintains scapular stability and upward rotation during overhead movements. Proper function prevents winging and shoulder impingement, enabling smooth, controlled pressing motion and joint integrity under load.

Q203. Answer: B

Explanation: Static stretching post-workout reduces muscle tension, enhances recovery, and maintains flexibility by promoting relaxation and increased blood flow. It's ideal after exercise when muscles are warm, aiding tissue restoration and minimizing soreness.

Q204. Answer: D

Explanation: Leading with the elbows and squeezing the shoulder blades activates the back muscles effectively, ensuring scapular retraction. This cue improves posture, enhances back engagement, and reduces reliance on biceps, fostering correct pulling mechanics.

Q205. Answer: B

Explanation: Maintaining a straight line from head to heels promotes neutral spinal alignment and core engagement during a plank. This position stabilizes the kinetic chain, prevents lower back sag, and maximizes the strengthening of deep core stabilizers for functional movement control.

Q206. Answer: B

Explanation: The plank activates deep core muscles, particularly the transverse abdominis and multifidus, which stabilize the spine and pelvis. This static exercise enhances neuromuscular control and spinal integrity, forming the foundation for efficient movement and injury prevention during dynamic activities.

Q207. Answer: C

Explanation: In the concentric phase of a lat pulldown, the scapula retracts and depresses as the latissimus dorsi shortens. This motion promotes proper shoulder mechanics, engaging the mid-back and avoiding excessive stress on the shoulder joint. Maintaining scapular control ensures safe and effective pulling strength.

Q208. Answer: B

Explanation: Cueing the client to keep their chest up and engage the core encourages upright posture and reduces forward trunk lean. This alignment activates the glutes and quadriceps properly while protecting the lower back and improving balance during lunging movements.

Q209. Answer: B

Explanation: The kneeling hip flexor stretch targets the iliopsoas and rectus femoris, effectively lengthening tight hip flexors. This stretch restores neutral pelvic alignment, enhances stride mechanics, and alleviates anterior pelvic tilt caused by prolonged sitting or repetitive hip flexion.

Q210. Answer: D

Explanation: Tempo dictates how long a muscle remains under tension during each contraction phase, influencing strength, endurance, and hypertrophy outcomes. Controlled tempo ensures form consistency, prevents momentum use, and enhances muscular control for safe, effective training progression.

Q211. Answer: B

Explanation: The latissimus dorsi is the prime mover during the seated row, responsible for shoulder extension and adduction. Proper scapular retraction ensures balanced back engagement, promoting postural stability and symmetrical upper-body development while minimizing strain on the lower back.

Q212. Answer: C

Explanation: Dynamic warm-ups enhance neuromuscular readiness by increasing heart rate, core temperature, and joint mobility. Controlled, movement-based activities such as lunges or arm circles prepare the muscles and nervous system for optimal force production and stability during training.

Q213. Answer: B

Explanation: The single-leg balance reach forward challenges balance in the sagittal plane by requiring anterior-posterior stability. It engages the glutes, core, and ankle stabilizers, improving control and coordination for forward-backward dynamic movements.

Q214. Answer: C

Explanation: Plyometric training develops explosive power by improving the rate at which force is generated. Exercises like jump squats and bounding utilize the stretch-shortening cycle, increasing neuromuscular efficiency and speed performance for athletic and functional activities.

Q215. Answer: C

Explanation: The knee push-up reduces resistance by shortening the lever arm, allowing proper form and strength development before progressing to full-body push-ups. This regression builds foundational upper-body endurance and core stability safely.

Q216. Answer: B

Explanation: Combining external and kinesthetic cues provides simple, actionable feedback that promotes better movement learning and control. This approach helps clients connect the desired motion with body awareness, improving execution without overwhelming technical jargon.

Q217. Answer: B

Explanation: The stability ball bridge enhances core stabilization endurance by engaging the glutes and deep trunk stabilizers while maintaining a neutral spine on an unstable surface. This promotes balance, control, and lumbo-pelvic alignment critical for functional strength.

Q218. Answer: A

Explanation: Inhaling before the lift and exhaling during the upward phase stabilizes intra-abdominal pressure, supporting spinal alignment and force transfer. This controlled breathing technique optimizes strength output and prevents excessive intra-thoracic pressure spikes.

Q219. Answer: C

Explanation: Maintaining an upright torso and tight core ensures proper balance and alignment during single-leg movements. This cue stabilizes the trunk, enhances proprioception, and minimizes compensations like knee valgus or forward lean.

Q220. Answer: B

Explanation: The rotator cuff stabilizes the shoulder joint by maintaining humeral head position during dynamic movement. This deep muscle group provides structural control, preventing impingement and supporting safe, efficient shoulder motion under load.

Q221. Answer: B

Explanation: The single-leg balance reach enhances proprioception by engaging neuromuscular pathways that control joint stability and spatial awareness. It strengthens small stabilizers in the ankle and hip, vital for coordination and balance development.

Q222. Answer: D

Explanation: Cable rotations strengthen the obliques and deep core muscles responsible for rotational stability in the transverse plane. This improves spinal control, athletic rotation efficiency, and functional trunk strength for sport and daily movements.

Q223. Answer: B

Explanation: Standing behind the lifter with hands near the rib cage allows immediate assistance if the lifter fails a rep. This position offers balanced support without obstructing the movement or altering bar path, ensuring safety during heavy squats.

Q224. Answer: B

Explanation: Dynamic stretching uses active movement patterns that progressively increase range of motion while maintaining muscular activation. It effectively prepares the neuromuscular system for performance by increasing mobility, blood flow, and coordination.

Q225. Answer: C

Explanation: The gluteus maximus drives hip extension during the step-up, providing power and stability. Proper activation ensures efficient movement mechanics and reduces strain on the lower back and knees by emphasizing posterior chain engagement.

Q226. Answer: B

Explanation: Controlled tempo and slow movement speed enhance neuromuscular engagement and stability. Slower execution challenges balance and proprioception, allowing improved control and coordination throughout dynamic stability exercises.

Q227. Answer: A

Explanation: Medicine ball rotational throws develop explosive core power by training the trunk to produce and transfer force rapidly through the transverse plane. This dynamic movement enhances athletic performance and rotational strength essential for sport and function.

Q228. Answer: B

Explanation: Drawing the navel in engages the deep core stabilizers, keeping the hips level and the spine neutral. This alignment optimizes lumbo-pelvic stability and enhances endurance of the transverse abdominis and obliques during static holds.

Q229. Answer: B

Explanation: The hip hinge pattern underlies proper kettlebell swing technique, engaging the glutes and hamstrings for powerful hip extension. Mastering this movement ensures efficient posterior chain activation and protects the lower back from excessive flexion.

Q230. Answer: A

Explanation: Performing exercises on a stability ball increases core activation and challenges joint stabilizers by introducing instability. This improves neuromuscular coordination, postural control, and balance, making it ideal for foundational and rehabilitation training phases.

Q231. Answer: C

Explanation: In the front squat, the barbell rests on the front deltoids and clavicles, allowing an upright torso and reducing lumbar stress. This position shifts emphasis to the quadriceps and core while maintaining a neutral spine. Proper placement ensures balance and efficient bar path during descent and ascent.

Q232. Answer: B

Explanation: Cueing the client to push through their heels promotes balanced weight distribution and proper posterior chain activation. This correction stabilizes the kinetic chain, maintains heel contact, and prevents forward lean, ensuring optimal squat depth and joint alignment.

Q233. Answer: C

Explanation: The stability ball push-up enhances dynamic shoulder stabilization by forcing the rotator cuff and scapular muscles to maintain control on an unstable surface. This strengthens joint integrity, improves proprioception, and enhances neuromuscular coordination essential for upper-body functional strength.

Q234. Answer: A

Explanation: Static stretching performed post-exercise helps relax muscles, increase range of motion, and aid recovery. Holding each stretch for 30 seconds or longer promotes tissue lengthening and alleviates tension after physical exertion, optimizing flexibility and recovery.

Q235. Answer: B

Explanation: The pectoralis major produces shoulder flexion and horizontal adduction, drawing the arms together during pressing movements. It is the prime mover in the bench press, generating force through coordinated contraction with the triceps and anterior deltoids for upper-body strength development.

Q236. Answer: B
Explanation: The cable woodchop targets the obliques and deep core muscles responsible for rotational control in the transverse plane. It strengthens the trunk's ability to resist and produce rotational forces, improving athletic movement efficiency and functional core power.
Q237. Answer: D
Explanation: Spotting at the wrists provides immediate control if the lifter loses stability during a dumbbell chest press. This position enables quick assistance without disrupting natural pressing motion, ensuring safety while allowing the lifter to maintain form and confidence under load.
Q238. Answer: B
Explanation: The transverse abdominis acts as a deep stabilizer, maintaining intra-abdominal pressure and spinal integrity under load. Engaging this muscle supports postural control, reduces shear stress on vertebrae, and enhances overall lifting efficiency in compound movements.
Q239. Answer: D
Explanation: Dynamic stretching involves moving joints and muscles through their full range with controlled momentum, promoting mobility and muscle readiness. This method warms up tissues, activates neural pathways, and enhances performance without reducing muscular power output.
Q240. Answer: D
Explanation: The back extension targets the erector spinae and gluteus maximus, reinforcing posterior chain endurance and spinal stability. This exercise enhances posture and reduces lower-back strain risk by strengthening muscles that maintain upright alignment during movement.
Q241. Answer: B
Explanation: Maintaining a neutral spine with core engagement protects the lower back by evenly distributing forces along the kinetic chain. This cue reinforces proper posture and stability, preventing compensatory movements that may lead to spinal stress or injury.
Q242. Answer: A
Explanation: The side plank challenges the obliques and transverse abdominis to resist rotational forces, improving anti-rotation strength. This exercise enhances core endurance and postural stability essential for maintaining spinal alignment under dynamic conditions.
Q243. Answer: A
Explanation: Progressing from bilateral to unilateral stance increases balance challenge by reducing base support. This enhances proprioceptive feedback and joint stability progressively, allowing controlled adaptation and minimizing fall risk.
Q244. Answer: A
Explanation: Tight latissimus dorsi limit shoulder flexion, causing compensatory lumbar arching during overhead movements. Addressing lat tightness with stretching restores full range and protects the spine from hyperextension during pressing activities.
Q245. Answer: B
Explanation: The eccentric phase lengthens the muscle under tension, promoting controlled deceleration and hypertrophy. This phase develops tendon strength, enhances stability, and contributes to balanced muscular development, reducing injury potential during explosive movements.
Q246. Answer: C
Explanation: The stability ball plank activates deep core stabilizers while engaging postural muscles to maintain alignment on an unstable surface. This enhances lumbo-pelvic endurance, improves balance, and strengthens neuromuscular coordination for functional movement control.
Q247. Answer: A
Explanation: Weak gluteus medius fails to stabilize the femur, causing the knee to collapse inward (valgus movement). Strengthening this muscle improves hip stability and knee alignment, reducing injury risk during unilateral lower-body exercises.

Q248. Answer: A

Explanation: The squat jump trains explosive lower-body power by rapidly generating and absorbing force through the stretch-shortening cycle. It strengthens fast-twitch fibers, improving performance in athletic and functional movements requiring speed and elevation.

Q249. Answer: B

Explanation: Circuit training alternates between upper and lower body or different muscle groups with minimal rest. This structure improves muscular endurance, aerobic conditioning, and time efficiency, providing both strength and cardiovascular benefits.

Q250. Answer: B

Explanation: The cat-cow stretch mobilizes the thoracic spine through controlled flexion and extension. It enhances spinal mobility, relieves stiffness, and improves posture by promoting fluid joint movement and coordination between the upper back and core.

Q251. Answer: D

Explanation: A spotter's primary role is ensuring safety by assisting only when the client loses control or reaches failure. This promotes client independence, maintains form integrity, and builds confidence while reducing injury risk during challenging lifts.

Q252. Answer: B

Explanation: Reactive core training enhances the core's ability to stabilize rapidly in response to movement or external force. It strengthens neuromuscular coordination for explosive transitions, critical in sports requiring quick directional or rotational changes.

Q253. Answer: B

Explanation: Cueing "shoulders down and back" activates the lower trapezius and rhomboids while relaxing overactive upper traps. This promotes proper scapular retraction and depression, ensuring efficient pulling motion and joint safety.

Q254. Answer: A

Explanation: The single-leg balance reach improves ankle joint stability by engaging intrinsic foot muscles and lower-leg stabilizers. It enhances proprioceptive feedback, balance control, and coordination—key factors for reducing ankle sprains and improving movement precision.

Q255. Answer: B

Explanation: Proprioceptive Neuromuscular Facilitation (PNF) uses alternating muscle contractions and relaxations to enhance flexibility. The contraction stimulates the Golgi tendon organ, followed by relaxation allowing deeper stretch, effectively increasing joint range and muscle extensibility.

Q256. Answer: B

Explanation: Cueing the client to push their hips back while maintaining a neutral spine preserves posterior chain alignment and prevents lumbar strain. This movement pattern emphasizes hip hinge mechanics, activating the glutes and hamstrings while maintaining spinal integrity and maximizing safety during lifting.

Q257. Answer: C

Explanation: Training on a stability ball engages deep stabilizers like the transverse abdominis by challenging balance and proprioception. The unstable surface demands continuous muscular adjustment, improving core activation, spinal alignment, and neuromuscular coordination during dynamic or static movements.

Q258. Answer: A

Explanation: The concentric phase of the cable chest press involves shoulder flexion and horizontal adduction, primarily driven by the pectoralis major. This coordinated movement pushes the load forward efficiently, emphasizing chest activation while maintaining joint stability and control through proper alignment.

Q259. Answer: B

Explanation: The single-leg Romanian deadlift challenges the body to maintain balance and postural alignment through dynamic movement. It strengthens stabilizers across the hip, core, and ankle while improving proprioception and neuromuscular coordination essential for functional control.

Q260. Answer: B

Explanation: Effective cueing improves movement quality and ensures exercises are performed safely with correct technique. It reinforces optimal joint alignment, muscle activation, and kinetic chain coordination, preventing compensations that could lead to injury and maximizing exercise effectiveness for long-term results.

Q261. Answer: B

Explanation: The Stabilization Endurance phase emphasizes neuromuscular control, postural alignment, and joint stability. By using controlled tempos and unstable environments, it teaches proper movement patterns and core engagement before progressing to higher load or velocity training.

Q262. Answer: C

Explanation: The Strength Endurance phase in the OPT model generally uses 8–12 repetitions at moderate loads. This range develops muscular endurance while reinforcing prime mover strength, bridging the gap between stabilization and hypertrophy phases.

Q263. Answer: B

Explanation: Tempo defines the duration of each movement phase—eccentric, isometric, and concentric—directly influencing time under tension. Controlled tempos enhance stability and muscular adaptation by improving coordination and technique precision across training phases.

Q264. Answer: C

Explanation: The Power phase emphasizes maximal velocity and explosive movement. This increases the rate of force production by combining strength and speed through exercises like jump squats or medicine ball throws. Fast tempo enhances dynamic performance and neuromuscular reactivity.

Q265. Answer: C

Explanation: Rest intervals of 3–5 minutes allow complete recovery of ATP–PC energy stores during maximal strength training. This ensures high performance across sets and promotes optimal neuromuscular adaptation for maximal force output.

Q266. Answer: B

Explanation: Circuit training alternates exercises targeting different body regions with minimal rest, improving both muscular endurance and cardiovascular conditioning. It efficiently manages training time while enhancing metabolic demand.

Q267. Answer: C

Explanation: Power training in the OPT model combines a heavy strength exercise (e.g., squats) with a biomechanically similar power movement (e.g., jump squats). This pairing enhances both force and velocity to optimize the rate of force production.

Q268. Answer: A

Explanation: The Hypertrophy phase focuses on muscular enlargement through moderate-to-high volume and controlled intensity. Increased time under tension stimulates myofibrillar growth and improves metabolic stress, promoting overall muscle mass development.

Q269. Answer: B

Explanation: Beginners benefit from 2–3 nonconsecutive training days per week, allowing sufficient recovery and adaptation. This schedule builds consistency, promotes neuromuscular learning, and reduces the risk of overtraining or injury.

Q270. Answer: D

Explanation: Undulating periodization alternates training variables frequently to prevent adaptation plateaus. By varying intensity and volume, it maintains progression, improves multiple fitness qualities, and sustains motivation through dynamic programming.

Q271. Answer: B
Explanation: Progression in the OPT model depends on a client's individual adaptation level. Trainers adjust load, volume, and complexity based on current performance and readiness to ensure continual improvement and prevent injury.
Q272. Answer: B
Explanation: Stabilization Endurance training uses 2–3 sets per exercise with lighter loads and higher reps. This volume supports endurance, balance, and control while minimizing fatigue, preparing clients for more demanding strength phases.
Q273. Answer: C
Explanation: The Maximal Strength phase focuses on lifting near-maximal loads for low repetitions to increase neural recruitment and force output. It enhances overall lifting capacity, forming a foundation for power development.
Q274. Answer: B
Explanation: Free weights and body weight exercises enhance joint stability and proprioception, aligning with the Stabilization Endurance goal. They challenge core control and kinetic chain coordination under manageable loads.
Q275. Answer: A
Explanation: Short rest intervals of 0–60 seconds maintain metabolic stress and increase muscle pump, stimulating hypertrophic growth. Limited recovery promotes cellular adaptation and encourages anabolic hormone release.
Q276. Answer: A
Explanation: Volume represents the total workload (sets × reps × load). It quantifies training stress and influences adaptation. Adjusting volume ensures proper progression and recovery across training cycles.
Q277. Answer: B
Explanation: Strength Endurance training pairs a traditional strength exercise with a stability-focused movement. This combination enhances endurance while reinforcing proper form and muscle coordination across integrated systems.
Q278. Answer: C
Explanation: The Power phase emphasizes generating force rapidly through high-velocity exercises. It develops neuromuscular efficiency and performance potential by integrating heavy and explosive training modalities.
Q279. Answer: B
Explanation: The medicine ball slam trains explosive power by utilizing the stretch-shortening cycle. It enhances full-body coordination and the ability to generate and absorb force rapidly, translating to athletic performance improvements.
Q280. Answer: B
Explanation: Strength Endurance training bridges stabilization and strength by improving prime mover endurance under resistance. It enhances postural alignment and movement efficiency, essential for progression to more intense phases.
Q281. Answer: C
Explanation: Performing 12–20 repetitions per set targets muscular endurance by emphasizing prolonged contraction and low-to-moderate loads. This enhances stamina and improves the ability to sustain submaximal force.
Q282. Answer: A
Explanation: The 4/2/1 tempo promotes controlled eccentric and isometric phases, enhancing neuromuscular control and stability. It helps correct imbalances and strengthens connective tissue integrity during foundational training.
Q283. Answer: C

Explanation: Power training requires 3–5 minutes of rest to replenish ATP–PC stores, ensuring full recovery for maximal explosive performance. Adequate rest sustains high velocity and force production across sets.

Q284. Answer: D

Explanation: The Maximal Strength phase uses high intensity (85–100% 1RM) for 4–6 reps across multiple sets. This structure enhances neural activation and muscular recruitment for peak strength capacity.

Q285. Answer: C

Explanation: The pyramid system progressively increases and decreases load within a session, stimulating varied muscle fiber recruitment. This intensity variation promotes muscular growth through metabolic and mechanical overload.

Q286. Answer: C

Explanation: Advanced athletes can train 4–6 days per week during the Power phase, as their recovery capacity and adaptation readiness allow higher frequency and intensity, enhancing peak force and velocity development.

Q287. Answer: A

Explanation: Hypertrophy training utilizes the highest volume with moderate-to-high loads and short rest intervals. This extended workload maximizes muscle tension and metabolic stress, key drivers for muscular growth.

Q288. Answer: B

Explanation: Intensity directly determines the primary adaptation—strength, endurance, or power. Adjusting load relative to 1RM aligns training stimulus with specific performance or physique goals.

Q289. Answer: B

Explanation: Pairing a strength move (squat) with a biomechanically similar explosive action (jump squat) aligns with Power phase superset principles, enhancing the rate of force production through post-activation potentiation.

Q290. Answer: A

Explanation: Short rest periods of 0–60 seconds between supersets sustain heart rate and endurance while maintaining strength intensity. This supports metabolic conditioning and muscular control.

Q291. Answer: C

Explanation: Beginning with multi-joint, compound exercises ensures maximal energy for demanding lifts and promotes efficient neuromuscular recruitment. Isolation exercises follow to refine specific muscles.

Q292. Answer: D

Explanation: Power training uses explosive tempos to enhance velocity and rapid force application. This stimulates high-threshold motor units, improving dynamic performance and reactive ability.

Q293. Answer: C

Explanation: Training at 75–85% of 1RM optimizes mechanical tension and time under tension for muscle growth. This intensity stimulates both slow and fast-twitch fibers, promoting hypertrophic adaptation.

Q294. Answer: A

Explanation: Maximal Strength training emphasizes lifting near-maximum loads for 1–5 reps, targeting neural adaptations and high-force output. This builds foundational strength for advanced power development.

Q295. Answer: A

Explanation: Power training integrates light-to-moderate loads with maximal velocity, developing rapid force production. This combination enhances movement efficiency and performance in explosive actions.

Q296. Answer: A

Explanation: Short rest periods of up to 60 seconds keep muscles under consistent stress, developing endurance and improving recovery efficiency. This method promotes cardiovascular and muscular conditioning simultaneously.

Q297. Answer: B
Explanation: The stability ball push-up challenges balance and core stability while limiting heavy load. It develops foundational neuromuscular coordination and kinetic chain control before advancing to heavier or complex lifts.
Q298. Answer: B
Explanation: Intensity corresponds to the percentage of 1RM used, dictating the training effect. Higher loads increase neuromuscular demand, driving strength and hypertrophy adaptations based on the desired goal.
Q299. Answer: B
Explanation: Active rest uses light activities like walking or yoga to enhance circulation, reduce muscle soreness, and accelerate recovery. It maintains mobility and readiness without adding fatigue or load stress.
Q300. Answer: B
Explanation: Periodization systematically varies training volume and intensity over time to maximize adaptation while preventing overtraining. It ensures progressive overload and structured recovery, optimizing performance outcomes safely.

Questions (301-400)

Q301. What is the primary goal of the stabilization phase in the OPT model?

A. Maximize muscle hypertrophy
B. Develop maximal strength
C. Improve neuromuscular efficiency and stability
D. Increase power output

Q302. Which acute variable should be increased first when progressing a client in resistance training?

A. Intensity
B. Volume
C. Frequency
D. Load speed

Q303. During the strength endurance phase, which type of resistance training system is most appropriate?

A. Single-set system
B. Circuit training
C. Superset system (strength + stabilization)
D. Pyramid system

Q304. What is the optimal repetition range for hypertrophy training according to the OPT model?

A. 1–5
B. 6–12
C. 12–20
D. > 20

Q305. Which training system alternates upper and lower body exercises to minimize rest time?

A. Peripheral Heart Action (PHA) training
B. Pyramid training
C. Split routine training
D. Compound set training

Q306. What adaptation results primarily from power-training phases?

A. Improved local muscular endurance
B. Enhanced maximal force production
C. Increased rate of force production
D. Improved postural stability

Q307. Which factor best determines resistance-training frequency for an experienced client?

A. Available gym equipment
B. Training intensity and recovery ability
C. Client's occupation
D. Preferred exercise types

Q308. In a four-week mesocycle, what is the main focus of week 4 (deload week)?

A. Testing maximal lifts
B. Reducing training load to aid recovery
C. Increasing intensity and sets
D. Adding new exercises

Q309. Which progression increases mechanical overload most effectively?

A. Decreasing rest periods
B. Switching exercise order
C. Reducing repetitions
D. Increasing load

Q310. What does the term "specificity" refer to in program design?
A. Targeting one muscle group repeatedly
B. Training adaptations mirror the type of stress imposed
C. Performing exercises randomly for variety
D. Using only high-intensity workouts
Q311. What is the correct order of exercise selection for an advanced client?
A. Isolation → Multi-joint → Power
B. Multi-joint → Power → Isolation
C. Power → Multi-joint → Isolation
D. Isolation → Power → Multi-joint
Q312. Which rest interval best supports maximal strength development?
A. 0–30 seconds
B. 30–90 seconds
C. 2–5 minutes
D. > 10 minutes
Q313. The "general adaptation syndrome" in program design describes:
A. Metabolic fatigue only
B. Progressive physical adaptation to stress
C. Nutritional changes with training
D. Emotional adaptation to exercise
Q314. Which training variable primarily drives endurance adaptations?
A. Load
B. Exercise type
C. Rest period
D. Repetition volume
Q315. What is the recommended repetition tempo for hypertrophy training?
A. 4-2-1-0
B. 2-0-2-0
C. 1-1-1-0
D. X-0-X-0 (explosive)
Q316. In linear periodization, intensity typically:
A. Remains constant throughout
B. Decreases as volume increases
C. Increases progressively as volume decreases
D. Fluctuates randomly week to week
Q317. Which training principle states that benefits are lost when training stops?
A. Specificity
B. Overload
C. Reversibility
D. Variation
Q318. What is the best exercise order for optimizing power output and safety?
A. Core → Assistance → Power
B. Power → Core → Assistance
C. Assistance → Power → Core
D. Isolation → Core → Power
Q319. What adaptation primarily results from training at 1–5 reps per set with 85–100% 1RM?
A. Hypertrophy
B. Muscular endurance

C. Maximal strength
D. Aerobic capacity

Q320. What is the main benefit of incorporating balance and core training into program design?
A. Improved isolation of major muscles
B. Enhanced kinetic chain stability and movement efficiency
C. Increased muscular size
D. Improved aerobic capacity

Q321. When designing a program for weight loss, which variable should be prioritized?
A. Load intensity
B. Total caloric expenditure
C. Rest duration between sets
D. Exercise order

Q322. What is the primary purpose of the warm-up phase in a session?
A. Burn calories before strength training
B. Enhance muscle hypertrophy
C. Induce fatigue before the main workout
D. Increase body temperature and neural readiness

Q323. Which type of exercise system involves completing all sets for one muscle group before moving to another?
A. Pyramid system
B. Horizontal loading system
C. Vertical loading system
D. Peripheral Heart Action

Q324. What is the recommended rest time between circuits in circuit training for endurance?
A. 0–30 seconds
B. 1–2 minutes
C. 3–5 minutes
D. 5–8 minutes

Q325. Which principle dictates gradual changes in training volume, intensity, and frequency over time?
A. Variation
B. Specificity
C. Overload
D. Reversibility

Q326. Which adaptation occurs primarily during the resistance development stage of the General Adaptation Syndrome?
A. Decreased strength levels
B. Improved performance and adaptation
C. Overtraining and regression
D. Acute fatigue and soreness

Q327. Which training variable should be decreased to allow optimal recovery in an overreaching program?
A. Load
B. Rest intervals
C. Volume
D. Intensity

Q328. When designing resistance training for older adults, the primary focus should be:
A. Maximal load lifting
B. Power output development

C. Functional strength and balance
D. Hypertrophy specialization

Q329. What is the primary purpose of periodization in program design?
A. Prevent adaptation
B. Ensure consistent overload and recovery cycles
C. Maximize random variation
D. Minimize training frequency

Q330. The "OPT model" primarily uses which type of periodization?
A. Reverse linear
B. Nonlinear (undulating)
C. Linear
D. Block

Q331. For an endurance athlete entering the strength endurance phase, what is the best rep range?
A. 1–5
B. 6–12
C. 12–20
D. >25

Q332. Which of the following best defines the term "training volume"?
A. Load multiplied by repetitions and sets
B. Total workout duration
C. Total rest time per session
D. Frequency of training sessions

Q333. What is the most effective rest interval for hypertrophy development?
A. 0–30 seconds
B. 30–90 seconds
C. 2–5 minutes
D. >6 minutes

Q334. During the strength phase, what is the optimal tempo for resistance exercises?
A. 4-2-1-0
B. 2-0-2-0
C. X-0-X-0
D. 1-1-1-1

Q335. Which principle describes the need to vary training stimuli to prevent stagnation?
A. Overload
B. Specificity
C. Variation
D. Progression

Q336. The "power phase" primarily combines which two training types?
A. Stabilization and balance
B. Strength and speed
C. Endurance and hypertrophy
D. Core and flexibility

Q337. In the OPT model, which training variable is decreased from the stabilization phase to the power phase?
A. Load
B. Repetition speed
C. Rest time
D. Volume

Q338. Which type of training incorporates several sets with gradually increasing loads and decreasing repetitions?
A. Pyramid system
B. Circuit training
C. Drop set
D. Peripheral heart action
Q339. What is the main goal of the functional strength phase in program design?
A. Maximize muscle size
B. Improve integrated movement efficiency
C. Increase cardiovascular endurance
D. Isolate specific muscle fibers
Q340. Which adaptation occurs when rest intervals are consistently shortened?
A. Increased maximal strength
B. Improved muscular endurance
C. Reduced metabolic stress
D. Decreased training density
Q341. What is the key determinant for selecting exercises in a strength program?
A. Equipment availability
B. Client's movement assessments and goals
C. Trainer preference
D. Client's aesthetic desire only
Q342. The "Principle of Overload" states that:
A. Training stress must exceed current capacity to elicit adaptation
B. Rest should exceed work intervals
C. Volume and intensity must always decrease together
D. Training must be random for adaptation
Q343. In designing a weekly microcycle, what is most critical for avoiding overtraining?
A. High load frequency
B. Adequate rest and recovery sessions
C. Increasing repetitions daily
D. Eliminating warm-ups
Q344. Which acute variable directly controls metabolic demand during resistance training?
A. Exercise order
B. Repetition tempo
C. Rest intervals
D. Load selection
Q345. Which energy system predominates during a 5RM heavy squat?
A. Phosphagen (ATP-PC)
B. Glycolytic
C. Oxidative
D. Lactic acid system
Q346. What is the best strategy for progressive overload in endurance training?
A. Add heavy resistance exercises
B. Gradually increase total training time or distance
C. Increase rest between sessions
D. Decrease training frequency
Q347. Which of the following represents an advanced method for developing maximal power?
A. Slow eccentric training

B. Plyometric supersets
C. Circuit training
D. Static holds

Q348. When training for muscular endurance, what intensity should typically be used?

A. 40–60% 1RM
B. 70–85% 1RM
C. 85–100% 1RM
D. 30–40% 1RM

Q349. What is the key benefit of alternating body-part training splits?

A. Maximizes local fatigue daily
B. Reduces systemic fatigue while maintaining volume
C. Prioritizes only upper-body strength
D. Limits recovery time

Q350. In undulating periodization, what changes frequently between workouts?

A. Training environment
B. Intensity and volume
C. Exercise type only
D. Session frequency

Q351. What is the primary goal of the strength endurance phase in the OPT model?

A. Maximize hypertrophy
B. Increase neuromuscular efficiency under load
C. Develop maximal power output
D. Improve flexibility

Q352. What is the ideal training frequency for beginners starting resistance exercise?

A. 1 day per week
B. 2–3 nonconsecutive days per week
C. 5–6 days per week
D. Daily full-body sessions

Q353. What type of resistance training is most beneficial for improving muscular power?

A. High-load, low-velocity training
B. Endurance circuits
C. Low-load, slow-velocity training
D. Moderate-load, high-velocity training

Q354. Which variable should be manipulated first to progress an untrained client?

A. Load intensity
B. Volume and exercise complexity
C. Repetition tempo
D. Equipment type

Q355. What is the most appropriate rep range to develop maximal strength?

A. 1–5
B. 6–12
C. 12–20
D. >25

Q356. In a superset system, how are exercises structured?

A. One exercise per muscle group
B. Two exercises performed back-to-back with minimal rest
C. Multiple sets of one exercise before switching
D. Random exercise order

Q357. Which training phase includes the highest total volume?
A. Stabilization
B. Strength endurance
C. Hypertrophy
D. Power
Q358. Which adaptation occurs with progressive increases in load over time?
A. Neural regression
B. Strength and hypertrophy improvements
C. Reduced coordination
D. Metabolic decline
Q359. The "law of diminishing returns" in resistance training refers to:
A. Rapid adaptation without limits
B. Slower progress as experience increases
C. Permanent plateau after six months
D. Equal progress across all phases
Q360. What is the correct rest period for power training exercises?
A. 0–30 seconds
B. 30–90 seconds
C. 2–5 minutes
D. 6–10 minutes
Q361. Which progression is most appropriate for an intermediate lifter improving stability?
A. Add unstable surfaces
B. Increase load immediately
C. Skip warm-up
D. Reduce total repetitions
Q362. What is the optimal sequence of program phases for general fitness clients?
A. Power → Strength → Stabilization
B. Stabilization → Strength → Power
C. Strength → Power → Stabilization
D. Random rotation weekly
Q363. What does the term "acute training variables" refer to?
A. Short-term hormonal changes
B. Immediate exercise variables like sets, reps, rest, and tempo
C. Long-term periodization plans
D. Nutritional protocols
Q364. What is the primary purpose of circuit training in program design?
A. Maximize power output
B. Combine strength and cardiovascular benefits efficiently
C. Reduce workload
D. Focus solely on hypertrophy
Q365. Which type of exercise should typically be performed first within a workout?
A. Isolation
B. Core stability
C. Multi-joint compound
D. Assistance
Q366. The key goal of hypertrophy training is to:
A. Improve power output
B. Increase muscle cross-sectional area

C. Enhance balance and stability
D. Develop cardiovascular fitness
Q367. Which program design factor best prevents overuse injuries?
A. Performing the same routine daily
B. Regularly rotating exercises and intensities
C. Training until failure each session
D. Avoiding rest days
Q368. Which is an example of a "complex" training method?
A. Light cardio after lifting
B. Performing static holds
C. Supersetting antagonist muscles
D. Performing a strength exercise followed by an explosive movement
Q369. Which physiological adaptation results from progressive overload?
A. Decreased mitochondrial density
B. Increased neural efficiency and muscle recruitment
C. Reduced contractile protein synthesis
D. Loss of flexibility
Q370. What does the term "macrocycle" describe in periodized training?
A. A single workout
B. A one-week microplan
C. A long-term annual training plan
D. A four-week recovery block
Q371. Which system uses ascending and descending loads within the same session?
A. Superset system
B. Pyramid system
C. Circuit system
D. Peripheral heart action
Q372. The purpose of a "microcycle" in periodized programming is to:
A. Outline daily or weekly training details
B. Set annual competition goals
C. Determine career-long training themes
D. Adjust nutrition only
Q373. What is the key focus when training special populations?
A. High-intensity overload
B. Individual safety and medical considerations
C. Equal workload to healthy adults
D. Neglecting contraindications
Q374. Which variable defines the total amount of work done in a training session?
A. Intensity
B. Volume
C. Tempo
D. Frequency
Q375. What adaptation occurs primarily when training intensity is increased progressively?
A. Enhanced neuromuscular recruitment
B. Reduced force capacity
C. Lower coordination ability
D. Increased fatigue only
Q376. What is the primary goal during the power phase of the OPT model?

A. Increase muscle size
B. Maximize rate of force production
C. Enhance balance and coordination
D. Improve flexibility

Q377. When designing a program for a client with limited recovery ability, what should be reduced first?
A. Exercise intensity
B. Total repetitions
C. Rest duration
D. Exercise frequency

Q378. What is the main benefit of alternating push and pull exercises in a workout?
A. Maximizes local muscle fatigue
B. Improves movement balance and recovery efficiency
C. Increases single-joint strength only
D. Reduces caloricpenditure

Q379. Which type of training phase emphasizes maximal muscle fiber recruitment at high loads and low volume?
A. Stabilization
B. Strength
C. Hypertrophy
D. Power

Q380. The optimal rest period between sets for hypertrophy training is:
A. 0–30 seconds
B. 30–90 seconds
C. 2–3 minutes
D. 5–6 minutes

Q381. What is the most critical factor to consider before increasing training intensity?
A. Client's nutrition
B. Movement quality and form consistency
C. Type of equipment used
D. Facility temperature

Q382. What is the main adaptation achieved from performing exercises at a slow tempo?
A. Improved rate of force production
B. Enhanced cardiovascular capacity
C. Increased time under tension for hypertrophy
D. Greater speed development

Q383. What type of periodization includes multiple changes in intensity and volume each week?
A. Linear
B. Undulating
C. Block
D. Reverse linear

Q384. In a resistance training session, which exercise order optimizes performance and safety?
A. Isolation → Power → Multi-joint
B. Power → Multi-joint → Assistance
C. Assistance → Power → Isolation
D. Randomized order

Q385. When designing a plan for weight management, what type of resistance training variable should be emphasized?
A. High load and long rest

B. High volume and minimal rest
C. Low volume and slow tempo
D. Single-set sessions

Q386. The principle of progression requires:
A. Gradual increases in training stimulus over time
B. Sudden large increases in workload
C. Fixed resistance and volume
D. Random variation weekly

Q387. What does the "SAID" principle state in training design?
A. Strength adaptation involves delay
B. Specific Adaptation to Imposed Demands
C. Sudden Adaptation of Intensity Design
D. Static Aerobic Intensity Development

Q388. For athletes focusing on maximal power, which combination is most effective?
A. Heavy strength + speed training
B. Stability + flexibility training
C. Endurance + mobility
D. Light circuit work

Q389. What is the main purpose of a cool-down phase in resistance training?
A. Increase load tolerance
B. Lower heart rate and promote recovery
C. Enhance power output
D. Improve explosive speed

Q390. Which variable should be prioritized for improving muscular endurance?
A. Load intensity
B. Total volume and short rest
C. Exercise order
D. Equipment type

Q391. When training for strength, the optimal repetition range is:
A. 1–5 reps
B. 8–12 reps
C. 12–20 reps
D. >25 reps

Q392. What is the main purpose of including a deload week in training?
A. Stimulate hypertrophy
B. Facilitate recovery and reduce accumulated fatigue
C. Increase volume significantly
D. Maintain constant overload

Q393. Which variable has the greatest effect on training intensity?
A. Load
B. Tempo
C. Rest interval
D. Frequency

Q394. The purpose of a fitness assessment before program design is to:
A. Eliminate variation in training
B. Prescribe random workouts
C. Increase immediate workload
D. Evaluate a client's current physical capabilities and limitations

Q395. Which training system alternates heavy and light days within the same week?
A. Split routine
B. Undulating periodization
C. Linear progression
D. Circuit training
Q396. What is the best strategy for maintaining long-term training adherence?
A. Maximal effort every session
B. Periodic variation and goal setting
C. Repetition of identical routines
D. Removing recovery phases
Q397. The "mesocycle" in periodization typically lasts:
A. 1 day
B. 1–4 weeks
C. 3–4 months
D. 1 year
Q398. What is the purpose of incorporating tempo variations in resistance training?
A. To control movement speed and influence muscular stress
B. To make workouts longer
C. To reduce exercise complexity
D. To standardize every lift
Q399. Which principle best supports long-term performance improvements?
A. Random training
B. Progressive overload with adequate recovery
C. Static workloads indefinitely
D. High-intensity sessions daily
Q400. What is the main purpose of resistance training for endurance athletes?
A. Maximize muscle hypertrophy
B. Improve neuromuscular efficiency and injury prevention
C. Replace aerobic conditioning
D. Decrease muscle tone

Answer keys and Explanations (301-400)

Q301. Answer: C
Explanation: The stabilization phase focuses on enhancing muscular endurance, coordination, and joint stability through controlled, low-load, high-repetition movements. This improves inter- and intramuscular communication, ensuring the kinetic chain functions efficiently under controlled tension, setting a foundation for subsequent strength and power development.
Q302. Answer: B
Explanation: Increasing training volume (sets × reps) safely enhances work capacity before advancing intensity. It allows muscles, joints, and connective tissue to adapt gradually. This progressive overload respects physiological adaptation principles, minimizing injury risk while promoting sustainable strength and endurance improvements.
Q303. Answer: C
Explanation: The strength-endurance phase blends heavy strength moves with stabilization exercises in superset format. This pairing challenges prime movers under load and reinforces postural control immediately afterward, enhancing muscular endurance and core stability simultaneously for improved functional strength.
Q304. Answer: B
Explanation: Hypertrophy adaptations occur best in the 6–12 rep range, using moderate to heavy loads. This range provides sufficient mechanical tension and metabolic stress to stimulate muscle fiber growth through increased cross-sectional area, optimizing both strength and aesthetic muscle development.
Q305. Answer: A
Explanation: PHA training alternates upper and lower body exercises in sequence, maintaining elevated heart rate and circulation between regions. This design enhances cardiorespiratory demand and caloric expenditure while promoting muscular endurance and efficient recovery between localized muscle groups.
Q306. Answer: C
Explanation: Power training enhances the neuromuscular system's ability to generate maximal force in minimal time. By combining heavy strength exercises with explosive movements, the nervous system learns to recruit motor units rapidly, improving athletic performance and dynamic functional ability.
Q307. Answer: B
Explanation: Intensity and individual recovery dictate how often sessions should occur. Higher intensity requires longer recovery due to greater muscular and nervous system stress. Balancing workload and rest optimizes adaptation while preventing overtraining and maintaining performance progression.
Q308. Answer: B
Explanation: A deload week intentionally lowers load or volume to promote physiological recovery and supercompensation. It prevents accumulation of fatigue, stabilizes performance, and enhances long-term adaptation by allowing tissue repair and nervous system restoration.
Q309. Answer: D
Explanation: Increasing load directly augments mechanical tension on muscle fibers, driving strength and hypertrophy adaptations. This overload challenges neuromuscular recruitment capacity and promotes structural remodeling, making it the most efficient progression variable when proper technique is maintained.
Q310. Answer: B
Explanation: Specificity means that physiological adaptations are highly dependent on the type, duration, and intensity of training stimulus. Training must mimic desired performance demands to ensure functional carryover and precise adaptation of the neuromuscular and energy systems.
Q311. Answer: C

Explanation: Power exercises require maximal neural output and coordination; thus, they're performed first when fatigue is minimal. Multi-joint strength moves follow, with isolation exercises placed last to target specific muscles safely after primary lifts are complete.

Q312. Answer: C

Explanation: Maximal strength training stresses the nervous system and phosphagen energy pathway, requiring 2–5 minutes for ATP-PC replenishment. Adequate rest preserves force output, enabling consistent high-load performance across sets for maximal neural and muscular adaptation.

Q313. Answer: B

Explanation: General adaptation syndrome (alarm, resistance, exhaustion) explains how the body responds to stress. Properly dosed training stress triggers the resistance phase, leading to strength gains and performance improvement while avoiding overtraining or regression.

Q314. Answer: D

Explanation: High repetition volume increases metabolic and mitochondrial adaptations that enhance fatigue resistance. This greater total work stimulates capillary density and oxidative efficiency, improving muscular endurance and overall stamina during prolonged physical activity.

Q315. Answer: B

Explanation: A moderate 2-0-2-0 tempo provides sufficient time under tension to maximize mechanical stress without excessive fatigue. It balances eccentric and concentric durations, optimizing protein synthesis and muscle growth while maintaining technical control.

Q316. Answer: C

Explanation: Linear periodization gradually raises intensity while reducing total volume over time. This structured progression develops foundational endurance early, then transitions toward peak strength and power, aligning recovery cycles with performance goals effectively.

Q317. Answer: C

Explanation: Reversibility means that without continual stress, physiological adaptations regress toward baseline. Maintaining consistent training stimuli sustains performance gains, as muscle fiber size, neural efficiency, and endurance capacity diminish rapidly during inactivity.

Q318. Answer: B

Explanation: Power exercises demand maximal neuromuscular coordination; thus, they should precede heavy core lifts and assistance work. Performing them early ensures fatigue doesn't compromise technique, maintaining force velocity efficiency and reducing injury risk.

Q319. Answer: C

Explanation: High-intensity, low-rep resistance training recruits maximal motor units, enhancing neuromuscular coordination and strength output. This training develops maximal voluntary contraction ability without necessarily producing significant hypertrophic growth.

Q320. Answer: B

Explanation: Balance and core exercises enhance neuromuscular control across the kinetic chain. This stability supports efficient movement mechanics, allowing safer and more powerful force transfer during complex strength and power exercises.

Q321. Answer: B

Explanation: Caloric expenditure governs fat reduction. Combining moderate resistance training with high total volume, shorter rest, and elevated heart rate maximizes energy use. This strategy promotes fat oxidation and sustainable weight management.

Q322. Answer: D

Explanation: A warm-up elevates muscle temperature, heart rate, and nervous system activation, improving joint mobility and coordination. These physiological changes enhance performance efficiency and reduce injury risk in subsequent high-intensity exercise.

Q323. Answer: B

Explanation: Horizontal loading requires finishing all prescribed sets of a specific exercise before proceeding. This allows greater focus on individual muscle performance, maximizing overload and technique consistency for targeted strength gains.

Q324. Answer: A

Explanation: Short rest intervals of 0–30 seconds maintain elevated heart rate and promote continuous oxygen demand. This approach enhances muscular endurance and aerobic conditioning by limiting full recovery between exercises within each circuit.

Q325. Answer: A

Explanation: Variation, or periodization, involves systematically modifying training variables to prevent plateaus and maintain adaptation. This strategic fluctuation promotes continuous neuromuscular progress and recovery, ensuring long-term performance improvement.

Q326. Answer: B

Explanation: The resistance development stage signifies the body's successful adaptation to repeated training stress. During this phase, physiological systems adjust by improving neuromuscular coordination, energy efficiency, and strength capacity, allowing higher performance output with less perceived effort under the same workload.

Q327. Answer: C

Explanation: Reducing total training volume (sets × reps) allows the body to recover from accumulated fatigue while maintaining intensity to preserve strength and power. This controlled reduction prevents overtraining while promoting supercompensation, enhancing long-term adaptation and athletic performance.

Q328. Answer: C

Explanation: Older adults benefit most from programs emphasizing functional strength, balance, and coordination to maintain independence and reduce fall risk. Prioritizing controlled, multi-joint, moderate-intensity movements enhances stability and daily functional capacity while protecting joint integrity and cardiovascular safety.

Q329. Answer: B

Explanation: Periodization structures training into phases that balance overload with recovery. This approach systematically manipulates intensity and volume, optimizing adaptation while preventing stagnation or overtraining. It ensures performance peaks at strategic times and maintains continuous physiological progress.

Q330. Answer: C

Explanation: The OPT model follows a linear periodization framework, progressing from stabilization to strength to power phases. Each phase builds upon the previous one, gradually increasing intensity while reducing volume, ensuring progressive overload and systematic adaptation toward performance goals.

Q331. Answer: C

Explanation: Performing 12–20 repetitions per set targets muscular endurance by sustaining low to moderate loads over longer durations. This high-repetition approach improves fatigue resistance and efficiency of slow-twitch muscle fibers, directly supporting endurance performance demands.

Q332. Answer: A

Explanation: Training volume is calculated as load × repetitions × sets, representing total work performed. Monitoring this variable allows precise control of training stress and adaptation, ensuring progressive overload without exceeding recovery capacity or increasing injury risk.

Q333. Answer: B

Explanation: Rest intervals of 30–90 seconds balance metabolic stress and partial phosphagen recovery, ideal for stimulating hypertrophy. This duration maintains sufficient fatigue to promote hormonal responses and mechanical tension necessary for muscle growth while allowing repeated effort.

Q334. Answer: B

Explanation: A controlled 2-0-2-0 tempo ensures proper technique and mechanical tension. It allows efficient force application during concentric and eccentric movements, maximizing muscle fiber recruitment while maintaining control under load, which enhances strength adaptations.

Q335. Answer: C

Explanation: Variation involves periodic changes in training intensity, volume, and exercise selection to sustain adaptation. By altering stimuli, it prevents neuromuscular and metabolic plateaus, ensuring continual progression while reducing the risk of overuse or mental fatigue.

Q336. Answer: B

Explanation: Power training merges strength with speed to maximize rate of force development. It involves pairing heavy-load strength exercises with explosive, high-velocity movements, improving the ability to exert force rapidly during athletic or functional performance tasks.

Q337. Answer: D

Explanation: As clients advance through the OPT phases, training volume decreases while intensity and complexity increase. Reduced volume prevents overtraining and enhances recovery capacity, allowing greater focus on neural activation and maximal power output development.

Q338. Answer: A

Explanation: The pyramid system progressively increases load and reduces repetitions, efficiently developing both strength and hypertrophy. This ascending intensity sequence enhances neuromuscular coordination, mechanical tension, and muscle recruitment while safely preparing the body for heavier loads.

Q339. Answer: B

Explanation: The functional strength phase targets the coordination of multiple muscle systems to improve movement efficiency across kinetic chains. This approach builds strength that directly translates to everyday and sport-specific actions through dynamic stabilization and force coupling.

Q340. Answer: B

Explanation: Shorter rest intervals maintain elevated heart rate and metabolic demand, improving muscular endurance. This promotes greater fatigue tolerance and oxidative capacity, allowing muscles to sustain repeated contractions effectively during extended physical activities.

Q341. Answer: B

Explanation: Exercise selection should align with movement assessments, functional deficits, and client-specific goals. This ensures relevance and safety while promoting the intended adaptations, such as correcting imbalances or optimizing performance based on identified needs.

Q342. Answer: A

Explanation: Overload drives adaptation by applying a training stimulus that exceeds habitual levels. The body responds by enhancing muscle strength, endurance, or power capacity, adapting to meet increased demands imposed during structured, progressive training.

Q343. Answer: B

Explanation: Rest and recovery allow physiological systems to repair and strengthen following training stress. Scheduled recovery within each microcycle preserves performance quality, prevents overtraining, and supports continued adaptation in both strength and endurance capacities.

Q344. Answer: C

Explanation: Rest intervals regulate metabolic stress and energy system engagement. Short rest promotes anaerobic glycolysis and endurance adaptation, while longer rest enables phosphagen recovery for maximal strength. Adjusting rest effectively targets specific training goals.

Q345. Answer: A

Explanation: The phosphagen system provides immediate ATP for high-intensity, short-duration efforts like a 5-rep max lift. It relies on stored creatine phosphate to rapidly regenerate energy, supporting maximal force production over a brief timeframe.

Q346. Answer: B

Explanation: Gradual increases in training time or distance extend aerobic workload safely, enhancing cardiovascular and muscular endurance. This progression builds capacity while minimizing injury risk, ensuring steady adaptation of energy systems and tissue resilience.

Q347. Answer: B

Explanation: Plyometric supersets pair heavy strength moves with explosive power exercises, training the stretch-shortening cycle. This enhances neuromuscular efficiency and the ability to produce force rapidly, key for improving athletic power and dynamic performance.

Q348. Answer: A

Explanation: Training at 40–60% of one-repetition maximum provides a manageable load for sustaining longer sets. This promotes increased capillary density, mitochondrial function, and fatigue resistance necessary for enhanced muscular endurance performance.

Q349. Answer: B

Explanation: Alternating training splits between muscle groups allows local recovery while maintaining total weekly training volume. This structure supports optimal performance and adaptation across all muscles without overwhelming systemic recovery capacity.

Q350. Answer: B

Explanation: Undulating periodization modifies intensity and volume across short cycles, such as daily or weekly variations. These frequent fluctuations maintain neural stimulation and prevent plateaus, promoting continual progress in strength, hypertrophy, and endurance simultaneously.

Q351. Answer: B

Explanation: The strength endurance phase trains muscles to maintain force output under fatigue. It enhances neuromuscular efficiency by combining heavy lifts with stabilization exercises, improving coordination, joint stability, and muscular endurance essential for performance consistency.

Q352. Answer: B

Explanation: Beginners benefit most from 2–3 weekly sessions with rest days between. This frequency allows neuromuscular adaptation and tissue recovery while preventing overuse injuries, ensuring gradual progression and adherence to a sustainable exercise routine.

Q353. Answer: D

Explanation: Power development requires moderate resistance lifted explosively. High-velocity contractions recruit fast-twitch fibers and train the nervous system to generate force rapidly, improving athletic performance and movement efficiency during dynamic tasks.

Q354. Answer: B

Explanation: Increasing volume or movement complexity first promotes safe adaptation for untrained clients. This approach builds muscular endurance and motor control before adding heavy loads, ensuring proper technique and minimizing the risk of injury.

Q355. Answer: A

Explanation: Low repetition ranges of 1–5 reps using high intensity (≥85% 1RM) optimize neuromuscular recruitment. This load level enhances maximal force output through improved motor unit synchronization and firing frequency without excessive fatigue accumulation.

Q356. Answer: B

Explanation: Supersets pair two exercises performed consecutively, minimizing rest between. This method increases training density, saves time, and enhances muscular endurance or hypertrophy depending on exercise selection and intensity balance.

Q357. Answer: C

Explanation: The hypertrophy phase uses moderate to high loads across multiple sets and repetitions, creating the greatest total training volume. Sustained mechanical tension and metabolic stress stimulate muscle fiber growth and increased cross-sectional area.

Q358. Answer: B

Explanation: Gradually increasing resistance triggers greater recruitment of motor units and enhances muscle fiber size. This progressive overload strengthens both neural efficiency and structural adaptation, forming the foundation for continuous strength and performance development.

Q359. Answer: B

Explanation: As training experience grows, adaptations become harder to achieve due to physiological optimization. Advanced individuals require more specific and intense stimuli to progress, emphasizing the importance of variation and precise programming.

Q360. Answer: C

Explanation: Power exercises require near-maximal neural effort and phosphagen recovery. Resting 2–5 minutes between sets restores ATP-PC stores, ensuring each explosive repetition maintains maximal velocity and force output for optimal performance.

Q361. Answer: A

Explanation: Introducing unstable environments enhances proprioceptive demand and neuromuscular control. This controlled instability trains the body to stabilize under dynamic conditions, improving balance, joint integrity, and overall functional strength.

Q362. Answer: B

Explanation: Sequentially progressing from stabilization to strength to power develops foundational control before advanced intensity. This systematic approach ensures safe adaptation, balanced muscular development, and optimal transfer of training to functional performance.

Q363. Answer: B

Explanation: Acute variables are modifiable components within a single session, including sets, reps, tempo, rest, and load. Adjusting these parameters dictates training intensity, volume, and adaptation type for targeted performance outcomes.

Q364. Answer: B

Explanation: Circuit training alternates exercises with minimal rest, maintaining elevated heart rate while providing resistance benefits. This format efficiently enhances muscular endurance, caloric expenditure, and cardiovascular conditioning within a compact timeframe.

Q365. Answer: C

Explanation: Multi-joint compound exercises engage large muscle groups and require maximal coordination. Performing them first ensures energy and focus are highest, maximizing force output and safety before smaller, more fatigable muscle groups are trained.

Q366. Answer: B

Explanation: Hypertrophy training focuses on enlarging muscle fibers through mechanical tension and metabolic stress. This adaptation results in greater contractile protein synthesis and visible muscular growth, improving both performance and physique aesthetics.

Q367. Answer: B

Explanation: Varying exercises, loads, and rest intervals distributes stress across different joints and tissues. This strategic variation minimizes repetitive strain, supports recovery, and maintains steady performance without compromising structural integrity.

Q368. Answer: D

Explanation: Complex training pairs a heavy resistance exercise with a biomechanically similar plyometric movement, enhancing post-activation potentiation. This method boosts neural activation and power output by exploiting heightened motor unit readiness following heavy lifting.

Q369. Answer: B

Explanation: Gradual overload challenges the neuromuscular system to activate more motor units and synchronize contractions efficiently. This neural adaptation, combined with muscular strengthening, improves overall force production and athletic capability.

Q370. Answer: C

Explanation: A macrocycle represents the largest periodization phase, typically spanning several months to a year. It encompasses all mesocycles and microcycles, outlining progression toward long-term performance or competition goals.

Q371. Answer: B

Explanation: Pyramid training manipulates load and repetition count within one exercise, ascending to heavy loads then descending back. This dual pattern effectively targets both strength and endurance fibers, maximizing muscle recruitment and adaptive stimulus.

Q372. Answer: A

Explanation: Microcycles break down mesocycles into detailed weekly or daily plans. They specify exercise selection, intensity, and recovery scheduling, ensuring short-term structure aligns with long-term performance objectives and progression continuity.

Q373. Answer: B

Explanation: Programs for special populations must prioritize safety, medical conditions, and contraindications. Individualized adjustments in intensity, volume, and exercise type ensure effective, safe adaptations without exacerbating health risks or limitations.

Q374. Answer: B

Explanation: Volume quantifies total workload by combining sets, reps, and load across exercises. It determines the overall training stimulus, directly influencing muscle adaptation, energy expenditure, and recovery requirements.

Q375. Answer: A

Explanation: Increasing intensity challenges the nervous system to recruit more motor units at higher firing rates. This adaptation strengthens neural drive, improving maximal force production, coordination, and efficiency in high-load movement execution.

Q376. Answer: B

Explanation: The power phase focuses on training the neuromuscular system to exert maximum force in the shortest time possible. By combining heavy-load and explosive movements, it improves neural efficiency and muscle synchronization for rapid, powerful actions in athletic performance.

Q377. Answer: D

Explanation: Reducing training frequency allows the client more recovery time between sessions while maintaining quality and intensity. This adjustment ensures proper adaptation and prevents overtraining, maintaining progress without overwhelming recovery systems.

Q378. Answer: B

Explanation: Alternating push and pull exercises balances agonist and antagonist muscle development while providing local recovery for each group. This approach enhances symmetry, prevents overuse, and allows greater overall workload efficiency within a single session.

Q379. Answer: B

Explanation: The strength phase emphasizes lifting heavy loads at lower volumes to recruit high-threshold motor units. This develops maximal force output by enhancing neuromuscular coordination, increasing muscle fiber activation, and optimizing mechanical efficiency.

Q380. Answer: B

Explanation: A rest interval of 30–90 seconds balances metabolic stress and partial phosphagen recovery. This timing maintains muscle tension and hormonal response, creating the ideal environment for muscle growth through mechanical overload and metabolic fatigue.

Q381. Answer: B

Explanation: Ensuring correct technique and movement control prevents injury when increasing load or complexity. Quality of movement demonstrates adequate neuromuscular readiness to handle greater intensity, making it the key prerequisite for safe and effective progression.

Q382. Answer: C

Explanation: Slower tempos prolong time under tension, increasing mechanical stress on muscles. This stimulates greater metabolic buildup and protein synthesis, making it highly effective for promoting muscular hypertrophy and endurance within controlled movement patterns.

Q383. Answer: B

Explanation: Undulating periodization alternates training focus throughout the week, such as power, strength, and endurance days. This frequent variation maintains adaptation stimulus, preventing plateaus while promoting simultaneous improvement across multiple performance domains.

Q384. Answer: B

Explanation: Power movements require maximum neural activation and coordination, so they come first. Multi-joint compound lifts follow, targeting larger muscles while energy is still high. Assistance and isolation exercises conclude the session to refine specific areas safely.

Q385. Answer: B

Explanation: High-volume, low-rest resistance training elevates heart rate and caloric expenditure. It creates greater metabolic demand, boosting post-exercise oxygen consumption and fat oxidation, making it ideal for improving body composition and supporting weight loss goals.

Q386. Answer: A

Explanation: Gradual workload increases ensure continuous adaptation while minimizing injury risk. This structured progression enhances performance, allowing physiological systems to adjust efficiently without overtraining, forming the core of safe and effective long-term program design.

Q387. Answer: B

Explanation: The SAID principle explains that the body adapts specifically to the stress it experiences. Training programs must replicate the desired movement patterns, intensity, and energy systems to ensure the most relevant physiological and performance improvements.

Q388. Answer: A

Explanation: Combining maximal strength and high-velocity movements develops both force and speed capacities. This synergy enhances rate of force development, critical for explosive power performance such as sprinting, jumping, or throwing activities.

Q389. Answer: B

Explanation: The cool-down gradually reduces heart rate, promotes venous return, and aids removal of metabolic byproducts. It facilitates recovery and flexibility, preparing the body for subsequent sessions while minimizing post-exercise stiffness and cardiovascular stress.

Q390. Answer: B

Explanation: High total volume combined with brief rest intervals enhances local muscular endurance. Sustained workloads under partial fatigue increase mitochondrial efficiency and capillary density, improving the muscle's capacity for prolonged, repeated contractions.

Q391. Answer: A

Explanation: Lifting heavy loads for 1–5 repetitions targets maximal motor unit recruitment and neural efficiency. This intensity improves maximal force output and coordination, building foundational strength that supports all other training phases.

Q392. Answer: B

Explanation: A deload week allows physiological and neural recovery from accumulated training stress. It maintains adaptation while preventing overtraining, ensuring long-term progression by rebalancing fatigue, hormone levels, and central nervous system readiness.

Q393. Answer: A

Explanation: Load directly determines resistance intensity. Increasing weight elevates muscular tension, mechanical stress, and neural activation, which are essential for improving strength and power. It's the most influential variable controlling training intensity outcomes.

Q394. Answer: D

Explanation: Fitness assessments establish baseline data on strength, flexibility, balance, and cardiovascular health. Understanding current capabilities and limitations ensures individualized, safe, and effective programming aligned with the client's goals and readiness level.

Q395. Answer: B

Explanation: Undulating periodization alternates intensities within short timeframes, such as heavy, moderate, and light sessions weekly. This maintains varied neuromuscular stimuli, prevents stagnation, and promotes simultaneous improvements across strength, hypertrophy, and endurance.

Q396. Answer: B

Explanation: Regularly adjusting programming and setting achievable goals keeps clients motivated and engaged. Variety prevents mental fatigue and physical plateaus, while goal progression sustains consistency, ensuring steady long-term results and adherence.

Q397. Answer: C

Explanation: A mesocycle spans several months and represents an intermediate training block focusing on specific adaptations. It bridges the macrocycle and microcycle levels, aligning structured short-term progress with long-term performance targets effectively.

Q398. Answer: A

Explanation: Varying repetition tempo manipulates mechanical tension and time under tension, directly affecting muscular adaptation. Controlling movement speed enhances exercise specificity, reinforces proper technique, and targets endurance, strength, or hypertrophy outcomes accordingly.

Q399. Answer: B

Explanation: Continuous progress depends on systematically increasing stress while allowing recovery for adaptation. This balance strengthens both physiological and neurological systems, enabling consistent improvements in performance, resilience, and strength capacity.

Q400. Answer: B

Explanation: Resistance training enhances neuromuscular coordination, stability, and strength endurance, which improves running economy and reduces injury risk. It complements endurance work by strengthening connective tissue and improving movement efficiency for sustained performance.

Questions (401-500)

Q401. What is the main purpose of the warm-up before resistance training?

A. To fatigue muscles before heavy lifting
B. To increase heart rate, blood flow, and joint mobility
C. To test maximum strength
D. To burn extra calories

Q402. In resistance training, "time under tension" primarily affects which adaptation?

A. Muscular endurance
B. Coordination
C. Power
D. Hypertrophy

Q403. What is the best approach for progressive overload in hypertrophy training?

A. Drastically increasing weight every session
B. Gradually adding small increments in load or volume
C. Changing exercises daily
D. Reducing rest intervals to zero

Q404. Which variable should be modified first to increase total workload safely?

A. Rest period
B. Volume (sets × reps)
C. Intensity
D. Exercise selection

Q405. What is the key goal of the stabilization endurance phase?

A. Maximize muscle size
B. Increase maximal force production
C. Improve joint stability and postural control
D. Enhance anaerobic power

Q406. Which adaptation results from high-intensity, low-repetition training?

A. Improved cardiovascular endurance
B. Maximal strength development
C. Increased flexibility
D. Enhanced hypertrophy

Q407. When programming resistance training for fat loss, which element should be emphasized?

A. Short rest and compound movements
B. Long rest and isolation exercises
C. Minimal sets
D. Single-joint movements only

Q408. What is the primary adaptation from plyometric training?

A. Muscular endurance
B. Rate of force production
C. Cardiovascular conditioning
D. Flexibility

Q409. What does the term "training density" describe?

A. Total number of workouts per week
B. Session duration only
C. Load per repetition
D. Work performed relative to rest time

Q410. Which of the following best describes "functional strength"?

A. Isolating muscles for appearance
B. Strength expressed through coordinated, multi-joint movements
C. Lifting the heaviest possible load
D. Performing movements slowly under light resistance

Q411. Which phase of the OPT model focuses most on developing hypertrophy?
A. Stabilization
B. Strength endurance
C. Hypertrophy
D. Power

Q412. In the power phase, how should exercises typically be paired?
A. Two isolation movements
B. One strength exercise followed by one explosive exercise
C. Two endurance exercises
D. One flexibility exercise with one balance exercise

Q413. What is the correct definition of "training frequency"?
A. Number of repetitions per set
B. Number of training sessions per week
C. Number of exercises per session
D. Duration of each workout

Q414. Which exercise sequence is most appropriate for a strength-focused session?
A. Isolation → Power → Compound
B. Power → Compound → Isolation
C. Random order
D. Isolation → Compound → Power

Q415. Which adaptation occurs from combining resistance training with cardiovascular conditioning?
A. Reduced muscular strength
B. Slower recovery rate
C. Loss of lean mass
D. Improved metabolic efficiency and endurance

Q416. Which principle supports designing programs based on individual needs?
A. Specificity
B. Individualization
C. Overload
D. Reversibility

Q417. Which training system involves completing all sets for one exercise before moving to the next?
A. Circuit
B. Horizontal loading
C. Vertical loading
D. Superset

Q418. What is the most critical consideration when programming for special populations?
A. Increasing exercise complexity
B. Managing intensity based on health status
C. Reducing recovery periods
D. Avoiding multi-joint movements

Q419. Which method is most effective for developing maximal power in advanced clients?
A. Heavy strength paired with explosive movement
B. Low-load, slow-velocity work
C. Circuit training only

D. Isometric contractions
Q420. What is the key characteristic of block periodization?
A. Training multiple abilities simultaneously
B. Concentrating on one performance quality per cycle
C. Using the same load weekly
D. Eliminating recovery weeks
Q421. What is the primary role of carbohydrates in exercise performance?
A. Build muscle tissue
B. Provide immediate energy for working muscles
C. Aid in fat metabolism only
D. Maintain hydration balance
Q422. Which macronutrient provides the highest energy per gram?
A. Carbohydrate
B. Protein
C. Fat
D. Alcohol
Q423. What is the recommended protein intake for a general fitness client?
A. 0.4–0.6 g/kg
B. 0.8–1.0 g/kg
C. 1.2–2.0 g/kg
D. 2.5–3.0 g/kg
Q424. Which nutrient is essential for transporting oxygen in the blood?
A. Iron
B. Zinc
C. Vitamin D
D. Calcium
Q425. What percentage of total daily calories should come from carbohydrates for most adults?
A. 10–20%
B. 25–35%
C. 45–65%
D. 70–80%
Q426. Which vitamin plays a key role in calcium absorption and bone health?
A. Vitamin C
B. Vitamin D
C. Vitamin A
D. Vitamin K
Q427. What is the primary function of dietary protein?
A. Energy production only
B. Hormone synthesis and tissue repair
C. Hydration regulation
D. Electrolyte balance
Q428. Which of the following is considered a complete protein source?
A. Peanut butter
B. Brown rice
C. Eggs
D. Almonds
Q429. Which mineral is most involved in maintaining fluid balance during exercise?
A. Potassium

B. Phosphorus
C. Magnesium
D. Sulfur

Q430. What is the approximate caloric equivalent of 1 pound of body fat?

A. 2,000 kcal
B. 2,500 kcal
C. 3,500 kcal
D. 4,500 kcal

Q431. What type of carbohydrate is stored in the muscles and liver for energy use?

A. Glucose
B. Sucrose
C. Lactose
D. Glycogen

Q432. Which macronutrient has the greatest thermic effect of food (TEF)?

A. Carbohydrates
B. Proteins
C. Fats
D. Alcohol

Q433. Which vitamin is essential for collagen formation and immune support?

A. Vitamin A
B. Vitamin B6
C. Vitamin C
D. Vitamin E

Q434. What is the recommended daily intake of water for most adults?

A. 0.5–1 L
B. 1–1.5 L
C. 2–3 L
D. 4–5 L

Q435. Which of the following best defines "energy balance"?

A. Equal intake and expenditure of calories
B. Eating less than energy burned
C. Overeating regularly
D. Reducing exercise to conserve energy

Q436. What is the main fuel source during low-intensity, long-duration exercise?

A. Carbohydrates
B. Proteins
C. Fats
D. Creatine phosphate

Q437. What is the minimum recommended carbohydrate intake for brain function?

A. 30 g/day
B. 50 g/day
C. 75 g/day
D. 130 g/day

Q438. What is the function of dietary fiber?

A. Builds muscle tissue
B. Aids digestion and supports gut health
C. Enhances glucose absorption
D. Increases protein synthesis

Q439. What type of fat should be limited to reduce cardiovascular disease risk?
A. Unsaturated fats
B. Omega-3 fatty acids
C. Saturated and trans fats
D. Medium-chain triglycerides
Q440. What nutrient primarily aids in muscle contraction and nerve transmission?
A. Calcium
B. Iron
C. Phosphorus
D. Fluoride
Q441. Which of the following foods is the richest source of omega-3 fatty acids?
A. Chicken breast
B. Salmon
C. Olive oil
D. Whole wheat bread
Q442. Which nutrient should be replenished first after endurance exercise?
A. Protein
B. Fat
C. Carbohydrates
D. Fiber
Q443. What is the role of sodium in the body?
A. Strengthens connective tissue
B. Maintains fluid balance and nerve signaling
C. Promotes muscle growth
D. Increases energy production
Q444. Which of the following best supports post-exercise recovery?
A. Consuming protein and carbohydrates within 30–60 minutes
B. Restricting fluids after activity
C. Consuming only fats
D. Skipping the meal after training
Q445. Which macronutrient provides the quickest source of energy during intense exercise?
A. Protein
B. Fat
C. Carbohydrate
D. Fiber
Q446. Which macronutrient is most important for repairing muscle tissue after resistance training?
A. Fat
B. Carbohydrate
C. Protein
D. Water
Q447. What is the primary function of dietary fat in the body?
A. Provide immediate energy for exercise
B. Insulate and protect vital organs
C. Enhance glycogen storage
D. Increase hydration levels
Q448. Why is hydration critical for exercise performance?
A. It increases protein synthesis directly
B. It decreases sweat rate

C. It prevents muscle hypertrophy
D. It enhances oxygen transport and thermoregulation

Q449. Which vitamin acts as a powerful antioxidant protecting cells from oxidative stress?
A. Vitamin D
B. Vitamin E
C. Vitamin K
D. Vitamin B12

Q450. What is the main energy system used during prolonged moderate-intensity exercise?
A. ATP-PC
B. Glycolytic
C. Oxidative (aerobic)
D. Lactic acid system

Q451. Which nutrient class includes compounds like starches and sugars?
A. Proteins
B. Carbohydrates
C. Lipids
D. Vitamins

Q452. Why is it important to consume carbohydrates with protein after intense training?
A. It promotes rapid fat oxidation
B. It enhances glycogen replenishment and muscle repair
C. It reduces total caloric intake
D. It suppresses water retention

Q453. What is the primary role of B vitamins in metabolism?
A. Provide direct fuel for muscles
B. Act as coenzymes for energy production
C. Build structural tissue
D. Store excess glucose

Q454. What is the best source of dietary calcium?
A. Citrus fruit
B. Green vegetables
C. Dairy products
D. Nuts and seeds

Q455. Which nutrient is most important for restoring glycogen after long-duration exercise?
A. Fat
B. Protein
C. Carbohydrate
D. Fiber

Q456. What is the main purpose of dietary guidelines for Americans?
A. Promote weight loss programs
B. Provide evidence-based recommendations for healthy eating patterns
C. Limit carbohydrate consumption entirely
D. Increase supplement sales

Q457. What nutrient deficiency is commonly linked to anemia and fatigue?
A. Zinc
B. Calcium
C. Iron
D. Sodium

Q458. What is the main function of water in temperature regulation during exercise?

A. Increases glycogen storage
B. Promotes heat dissipation through sweat evaporation
C. Stimulates energy metabolism directly
D. Lowers blood viscosity permanently

Q459. Which vitamin assists with calcium absorption in the intestines?
A. Vitamin D
B. Vitamin A
C. Vitamin C
D. Vitamin B12

Q460. What is the most energy-dense macronutrient?
A. Carbohydrates
B. Protein
C. Fat
D. Alcohol

Q461. What is the primary storage form of carbohydrates in the human body?
A. Glucose
B. Glycogen
C. Lactate
D. Fructose

Q462. What is the role of omega-3 fatty acids in human health?
A. Promote inflammation
B. Slow recovery after exercise
C. Increase LDL cholesterol levels
D. Reduce blood pressure and improve heart health

Q463. Why is protein timing important after resistance exercise?
A. It increases body fat oxidation
B. It enhances muscle protein synthesis and repair
C. It reduces hydration needs
D. It prevents glycogen storage

Q464. What nutrient plays the greatest role in maintaining osmotic balance and fluid distribution?
A. Phosphorus
B. Sodium
C. Chloride
D. Iron

Q465. Which vitamin is required for red blood cell formation and nervous system health?
A. Vitamin B12
B. Vitamin D
C. Vitamin A
D. Vitamin K

Q466. Which mineral works synergistically with calcium to strengthen bones?
A. Potassium
B. Phosphorus
C. Iron
D. Sodium

Q467. What is the main function of dietary antioxidants?
A. Increase oxidative damage
B. Neutralize free radicals and protect cells
C. Enhance water retention

D. Stimulate weight gain

Q468. Which nutrient combination most effectively promotes recovery after endurance events?

A. Fat and protein
B. Vitamins and minerals
C. Protein and carbohydrates
D. Electrolytes and water

Q469. What is the role of potassium in exercise physiology?

A. Promote energy storage as glycogen
B. Facilitate nerve conduction and muscle contraction
C. Decrease metabolic rate
D. Reduce water absorption

Q470. What is the best hydration guideline for athletes during exercise?

A. Drink only when thirsty
B. Consume small, regular amounts of water throughout activity
C. Avoid fluid intake until post-workout
D. Drink excessive volumes before starting

Q471. What is the primary function of glycogen in the human body?

A. Provide insulation
B. Serve as stored carbohydrate energy for muscles and liver
C. Maintain electrolyte balance
D. Promote fat metabolism only

Q472. What is the role of vitamin K in the human body?

A. Supports collagen formation
B. Enhances oxygen transport
C. Boosts energy metabolism
D. Facilitates blood clotting and bone metabolism

Q473. Which nutrient should be prioritized in hot and humid environments to prevent cramps?

A. Iron
B. Sodium
C. Vitamin D
D. Zinc

Q474. What is the primary function of dietary fiber in cardiovascular health?

A. Increases LDL cholesterol absorption
B. Reduces total and LDL cholesterol levels
C. Enhances triglyceride production
D. Raises blood pressure levels

Q475. What nutrient supports energy production in red blood cells by aiding oxygen transport?

A. Calcium
B. Iron
C. Phosphorus
D. Magnesium

Q476. What is the primary benefit of omega-3 fatty acids for athletes?

A. Enhance anti-inflammatory response and recovery
B. Decrease joint mobility
C. Increase muscle glycogen depletion
D. Raise LDL cholesterol

Q477. What is the function of phosphorus in the energy systems of the body?

A. Enhances glycogen breakdown

B. Contributes to ATP formation and energy transfer
C. Promotes fat oxidation directly
D. Maintains connective tissue strength

Q478. What is the main reason athletes should avoid dehydration during performance?

A. It causes faster glycogen synthesis
B. It increases cardiovascular strain and decreases endurance
C. It improves thermoregulation
D. It reduces muscle fatigue

Q479. What nutrient assists with the synthesis of DNA and cell division?

A. Folate
B. Vitamin C
C. Vitamin A
D. Vitamin D

Q480. What is the primary fuel for the brain and central nervous system?

A. Fat
B. Amino acids
C. Glucose
D. Ketones

Q481. Which macronutrient supports the absorption of fat-soluble vitamins?

A. Protein
B. Fat
C. Carbohydrate
D. Fiber

Q482. Why is meal timing important for athletic performance?

A. It limits hydration
B. It ensures nutrient availability for energy and recovery
C. It replaces the need for balanced nutrition
D. It prevents glycogen storage

Q483. Which mineral supports over 300 enzymatic reactions, including those in energy metabolism?

A. Zinc
B. Iron
C. Phosphorus
D. Magnesium

Q484. What is the key nutrient for preventing neural tube defects during pregnancy?

A. Vitamin C
B. Folate
C. Calcium
D. Iron

Q485. What is the main function of carbohydrates during high-intensity exercise?

A. Provide sustained low-energy output
B. Serve as the primary fuel for rapid ATP production
C. Support long-term fat oxidation
D. Replace water lost through sweat

Q486. Which nutrient supports the formation of connective tissue and wound healing?

A. Vitamin C
B. Vitamin D
C. Vitamin A
D. Zinc

Q487. What is the primary reason athletes need more protein than sedentary individuals?
A. To increase glycogen stores
B. To repair and rebuild exercise-induced muscle damage
C. To reduce fat oxidation
D. To maintain fluid balance
Q488. What is the best post-exercise carbohydrate intake strategy for glycogen resynthesis?
A. Consume small amounts 2–3 hours later
B. Consume 1.0–1.5 g/kg within 30 minutes post-exercise
C. Delay carbohydrate intake until next meal
D. Avoid combining with protein
Q489. What is the recommended percentage of daily calories from protein for active adults?
A. 5–10%
B. 10–15%
C. 15–25%
D. 30–40%
Q490. What is the importance of balanced macronutrient intake for general health?
A. Prevents muscle gain
B. Ensures optimal energy availability and physiological function
C. Reduces energy expenditure
D. Limits nutrient absorption
Q491. What is the most effective way to establish initial rapport with a new client?
A. Discuss personal achievements
B. Ask open-ended questions and actively listen
C. Immediately assign fitness goals
D. Use professional jargon to show expertise
Q492. Which communication skill involves summarizing what a client has said to confirm understanding?
A. Reflective listening
B. Questioning
C. Clarifying
D. Paraphrasing
Q493. According to the Transtheoretical Model, which stage describes a client considering change within six months?
A. Precontemplation
B. Contemplation
C. Preparation
D. Maintenance
Q494. What is the primary goal of motivational interviewing?
A. Convince the client to follow instructions
B. Help clients explore and resolve ambivalence toward change
C. Provide direct solutions to client problems
D. Focus only on goal achievement
Q495. Which question type best promotes client self-reflection and discussion?
A. Closed-ended
B. Leading
C. Open-ended
D. Yes-or-no
Q496. In the SMART goal framework, what does the "A" stand for?

A. Accurate
B. Attainable
C. Aggressive
D. Aligned

Q497. Which element of nonverbal communication can strongly affect client perception?
A. Tone of voice
B. Word choice
C. Email correspondence
D. Exercise demonstration

Q498. Which client-centered approach best increases self-efficacy?
A. Encouraging small, consistent successes
B. Providing constant external rewards
C. Using competitive motivation
D. Eliminating client input in decisions

Q499. What should a trainer do if a client expresses frustration about slow progress?
A. Dismiss the concern as normal
B. Reassess goals and provide encouragement
C. Increase workout intensity immediately
D. Ignore emotional feedback

Q500. What is the main purpose of reflective listening in coaching?
A. Repeat instructions clearly
B. Provide motivational feedback only
C. Directly challenge resistance
D. Demonstrate understanding and empathy

Answer keys and Explanations (401-500)

Q401. Answer: B
Explanation: A proper warm-up raises body temperature and enhances blood flow to working muscles, improving elasticity and joint mobility. This primes the neuromuscular system, improving performance while significantly reducing the risk of strains or injuries during training.
Q402. Answer: D
Explanation: Prolonging time under tension enhances muscle fiber recruitment and metabolic stress, which stimulate hypertrophy. The sustained load increases mechanical strain, initiating cellular signaling for muscle growth through greater protein synthesis and tissue remodeling.
Q403. Answer: B
Explanation: Incremental adjustments in load, sets, or repetitions provide a steady overload that encourages adaptation without overtraining. Gradual progression ensures consistent hypertrophic gains by balancing stress and recovery while maintaining proper movement mechanics.
Q404. Answer: B
Explanation: Increasing training volume allows for safe workload progression without abrupt intensity spikes. More sets or reps enhance endurance and conditioning while giving tissues time to adapt before adding heavier loads, promoting sustainable long-term progress.
Q405. Answer: C
Explanation: The stabilization endurance phase builds foundational strength by improving joint stability, core activation, and balance. Controlled, low-load, high-repetition exercises enhance muscular coordination and endurance, preparing the kinetic chain for heavier and more dynamic loads.
Q406. Answer: B
Explanation: Low-repetition, high-intensity training recruits fast-twitch fibers and optimizes neural efficiency, maximizing force production. This strengthens motor unit synchronization and firing rate, leading to measurable increases in overall maximal strength output.
Q407. Answer: A
Explanation: Compound exercises with short rest periods elevate heart rate and energy expenditure, maximizing fat oxidation. This strategy sustains high metabolic demand, increasing caloric burn during and after exercise while maintaining lean muscle mass.
Q408. Answer: B
Explanation: Plyometric training enhances the rate of force development by utilizing the stretch-shortening cycle. Explosive movements improve neural activation and muscle elasticity, enabling athletes to generate powerful contractions more efficiently in sports and functional tasks.
Q409. Answer: D
Explanation: Training density measures total work accomplished within a given time frame, balancing workload and recovery. Increasing density through shorter rests or greater volume enhances metabolic demand, promoting endurance and conditioning adaptations efficiently.
Q410. Answer: B
Explanation: Functional strength refers to the ability to apply force efficiently in coordinated, multi-joint movements. It integrates balance, stability, and mobility, allowing strength gains to transfer effectively to real-life or sport-specific actions.
Q411. Answer: C
Explanation: The hypertrophy phase specifically targets muscle growth by using moderate to high loads, 6–12 repetitions, and controlled tempo. This training induces both mechanical tension and metabolic stress, optimizing muscle fiber enlargement and density.
Q412. Answer: B

Explanation: Pairing a heavy strength exercise with an explosive power movement enhances neuromuscular coordination and post-activation potentiation. This method improves force velocity and prepares muscles to perform powerful, rapid contractions efficiently.

Q413. Answer: B

Explanation: Training frequency indicates how often a person performs workouts weekly. It determines cumulative workload and recovery balance, influencing overall adaptation rate and ensuring consistent progress aligned with individual goals and capacity.

Q414. Answer: B

Explanation: Starting with power exercises when energy levels are high maximizes neuromuscular output. Compound multi-joint movements follow to develop overall strength, and isolation exercises finish the session to refine specific muscle engagement safely.

Q415. Answer: D

Explanation: Integrating resistance and cardiovascular training enhances total energy metabolism and endurance. It improves oxygen utilization, muscle efficiency, and fat oxidation while preserving lean mass, contributing to overall conditioning and performance.

Q416. Answer: B

Explanation: Individualization ensures training programs align with each person's unique goals, fitness level, recovery rate, and biomechanics. It maximizes effectiveness by customizing exercise selection and volume to fit physiological and personal characteristics.

Q417. Answer: B

Explanation: The horizontal loading system completes all prescribed sets of one exercise before transitioning. This method focuses on strength and hypertrophy development, allowing concentrated effort and full recovery between sets for high-quality repetitions.

Q418. Answer: B

Explanation: Special populations require carefully controlled intensity that matches health status and medical considerations. Monitoring load, progression, and fatigue ensures safe training while enabling gradual improvements in strength, function, and overall fitness.

Q419. Answer: A

Explanation: Combining heavy resistance lifts with explosive movements trains both strength and speed capacities. This post-activation potentiation method enhances neural responsiveness and rate of force development, producing superior power output in advanced trainees.

Q420. Answer: B

Explanation: Block periodization isolates specific performance traits, such as strength, power, or endurance, in focused training blocks. This concentrated method optimizes adaptation by minimizing interference between competing physiological demands and enhancing peak performance outcomes.

Q421. Answer: B

Explanation: Carbohydrates serve as the body's main energy source during exercise, supplying glucose for muscle contraction. Stored as glycogen, they support high-intensity activity by maintaining blood glucose and delaying fatigue, ensuring consistent performance output.

Q422. Answer: C

Explanation: Fats yield approximately 9 calories per gram, making them the most energy-dense macronutrient. They serve as a critical long-term fuel source during low- to moderate-intensity activity and are essential for hormone production and cellular integrity.

Q423. Answer: C

Explanation: For most active individuals, consuming 1.2–2.0 grams of protein per kilogram of body weight supports muscle repair and adaptation. This range provides sufficient amino acids for recovery, growth, and maintaining lean body mass without excess intake.

Q424. Answer: A

Explanation: Iron is a crucial component of hemoglobin, allowing red blood cells to carry oxygen to tissues. Adequate iron levels enhance endurance and performance by supporting aerobic metabolism and preventing fatigue or anemia-related weakness.

Q425. Answer: C

Explanation: A balanced diet typically includes 45–65% of total calories from carbohydrates. This range supports optimal glycogen stores and energy availability for both daily activity and structured exercise without excessive caloric surplus.

Q426. Answer: B

Explanation: Vitamin D enhances intestinal absorption of calcium, supporting bone mineralization and structural strength. Adequate levels reduce the risk of osteoporosis and maintain muscle function, essential for performance and long-term musculoskeletal health.

Q427. Answer: B

Explanation: Proteins supply amino acids used for building enzymes, hormones, and tissue structures. They play a vital role in muscle repair and adaptation following exercise, supporting recovery, strength gains, and overall cellular maintenance.

Q428. Answer: C

Explanation: Eggs contain all nine essential amino acids in adequate proportions, classifying them as a complete protein source. This profile supports muscle recovery and protein synthesis, making eggs a highly efficient dietary protein option.

Q429. Answer: A

Explanation: Potassium regulates fluid balance, muscle contraction, and nerve transmission. It counteracts sodium's effects by helping retain intracellular fluid, supporting proper hydration and preventing cramps or fatigue during prolonged activity.

Q430. Answer: C

Explanation: One pound of stored fat equals roughly 3,500 calories. Creating a caloric deficit of this amount—through diet, activity, or both—generally results in one pound of fat loss over time, assuming consistent energy balance.

Q431. Answer: D

Explanation: Glycogen, the storage form of glucose, resides in muscle and liver tissue. It acts as a rapid energy reserve during exercise, fueling muscular contractions and maintaining blood glucose levels under physical stress.

Q432. Answer: B

Explanation: Protein digestion requires more energy than other macronutrients, resulting in the highest thermic effect. This increased metabolic cost supports satiety and contributes slightly to overall energy expenditure during digestion and metabolism.

Q433. Answer: C

Explanation: Vitamin C supports collagen synthesis, crucial for connective tissue integrity, and enhances immune function. It also aids in iron absorption, making it an important micronutrient for tissue repair and recovery processes.

Q434. Answer: C

Explanation: Consuming about 2–3 liters of water daily supports normal physiological functions and thermoregulation. Adequate hydration enhances nutrient transport, temperature control, and joint lubrication, preventing dehydration during daily and exercise activities.

Q435. Answer: A

Explanation: Energy balance occurs when caloric intake equals expenditure, maintaining body weight. Positive balance leads to gain, while negative balance results in weight loss. This concept forms the foundation for weight management strategies.

Q436. Answer: C

Explanation: During prolonged, low-intensity activity, fats serve as the predominant energy source. The oxidative metabolism of fatty acids provides sustained ATP production, conserving glycogen stores and supporting endurance performance efficiently.

Q437. Answer: D

Explanation: The brain relies heavily on glucose for energy, requiring about 130 grams of carbohydrates daily. This intake maintains cognitive function and prevents fatigue, ensuring sufficient glucose availability for neural and metabolic processes.

Q438. Answer: B

Explanation: Fiber promotes digestive health by improving bowel regularity and supporting beneficial gut bacteria. It slows glucose absorption, helping manage blood sugar and cholesterol levels while contributing to overall satiety and metabolic control.

Q439. Answer: C

Explanation: Saturated and trans fats increase LDL cholesterol and promote arterial plaque formation, elevating cardiovascular disease risk. Limiting these fats while emphasizing unsaturated sources supports heart health and circulatory efficiency.

Q440. Answer: A

Explanation: Calcium facilitates muscle contraction and nerve impulse transmission by triggering cross-bridge formation in muscle fibers. It also supports bone structure, making it essential for both skeletal health and neuromuscular function.

Q441. Answer: B

Explanation: Fatty fish like salmon provide high levels of omega-3 fatty acids, including EPA and DHA. These compounds reduce inflammation, improve cardiovascular health, and support cognitive function, making them vital for overall wellness.

Q442. Answer: C

Explanation: Replacing glycogen with carbohydrate intake post-exercise restores energy reserves and promotes recovery. Consuming carbohydrates immediately after endurance activity accelerates glycogen synthesis, enabling faster muscular recovery and readiness for subsequent sessions.

Q443. Answer: B

Explanation: Sodium helps regulate extracellular fluid balance and nerve conduction. It maintains osmotic pressure, enabling proper muscle contraction and hydration control, particularly critical during exercise when electrolyte losses are elevated.

Q444. Answer: A

Explanation: Combining carbohydrates and protein shortly after exercise replenishes glycogen stores and promotes muscle repair. This nutrient pairing accelerates recovery, enhances adaptation, and reduces muscle soreness by optimizing anabolic processes.

Q445. Answer: C

Explanation: Carbohydrates break down rapidly into glucose, supplying immediate ATP through glycolysis. This fast energy release supports high-intensity efforts, making carbohydrates essential for sprinting, lifting, and other anaerobic activities.

Q446. Answer: C

Explanation: Protein provides essential amino acids that repair damaged muscle fibers and stimulate muscle protein synthesis after resistance exercise. Adequate intake replenishes structural proteins and enzymes, allowing the body to adapt by increasing muscle size, strength, and resilience to future workloads. Without sufficient protein, recovery slows, and training adaptations become less efficient or incomplete.

Q447. Answer: B

Explanation: Fat serves multiple essential roles, including insulating the body, protecting organs, supporting hormone production, and aiding in the absorption of fat-soluble vitamins (A, D, E, K). While it contributes energy, its primary function is long-term energy storage and cellular structure protection. Adequate dietary fat maintains physiological balance, organ health, and efficient hormonal regulation.

Q448. Answer: D

Explanation: Proper hydration sustains blood volume, enabling efficient oxygen and nutrient transport to active muscles. It also supports thermoregulation by facilitating sweating and cooling, reducing the risk of heat stress. Maintaining fluid balance optimizes muscle contractions, cognitive focus, and endurance, allowing athletes to sustain performance intensity and delay fatigue during prolonged or intense exercise.

Q449. Answer: B

Explanation: Vitamin E protects cell membranes from oxidative damage by neutralizing free radicals generated during metabolism and intense exercise. This antioxidant function preserves cellular integrity, immune health, and tissue recovery. Adequate vitamin E intake supports longevity of red blood cells and prevents lipid peroxidation, a process that can impair muscle function and increase fatigue under stress.

Q450. Answer: C

Explanation: During moderate-intensity exercise lasting several minutes or longer, the oxidative or aerobic energy system predominates. It uses oxygen to break down carbohydrates and fats for ATP production, sustaining energy output efficiently. This pathway supports endurance by providing a steady energy supply, delaying fatigue, and promoting cardiovascular and metabolic adaptations essential for long-duration physical activity.

Q451. Answer: B

Explanation: Carbohydrates encompass simple sugars and complex starches that serve as the body's preferred energy source. They are broken down into glucose, fueling both the central nervous system and muscular contractions. Proper carbohydrate intake supports glycogen storage and blood glucose stability, ensuring sustained energy levels for exercise, cognitive performance, and overall metabolic efficiency throughout daily activities.

Q452. Answer: B

Explanation: Consuming carbohydrates with protein post-training accelerates glycogen restoration while stimulating muscle protein synthesis. Carbohydrates increase insulin levels, promoting amino acid uptake into muscle tissue, and protein provides the raw materials for repair. Together, they enhance recovery, reduce soreness, and prepare the body for subsequent sessions by optimizing nutrient availability and cellular regeneration processes.

Q453. Answer: B

Explanation: B vitamins serve as essential coenzymes that activate enzymes involved in carbohydrate, fat, and protein metabolism. They facilitate energy production by enabling nutrient conversion into usable ATP. Adequate intake supports optimal performance, neural function, and recovery, ensuring the metabolic pathways remain efficient under both resting and active conditions throughout physical training.

Q454. Answer: C

Explanation: Dairy products like milk, yogurt, and cheese provide highly bioavailable calcium essential for bone strength, nerve transmission, and muscle contraction. Calcium from these sources is efficiently absorbed, helping maintain bone mineral density and reducing the risk of osteoporosis. Regular intake also supports normal heart rhythm and muscular coordination during exercise and daily activity.

Q455. Answer: C

Explanation: Carbohydrates are the key nutrient for replenishing muscle and liver glycogen depleted during endurance activity. Rapid carbohydrate intake within two hours post-exercise maximizes glycogen synthase activity, restoring energy reserves for future sessions. This replenishment maintains performance consistency, prevents fatigue, and ensures full recovery for sustained training efficiency across repeated bouts of exercise.

Q456. Answer: B

Explanation: The Dietary Guidelines for Americans serve as a national framework to help individuals adopt nutrient-dense, balanced eating habits. They emphasize variety, moderation, and portion control to prevent chronic disease and promote overall health. These recommendations guide policy, nutrition education, and meal planning across all populations, ensuring accessible, science-based nutrition guidance for long-term wellness.

Q457. Answer: C

Explanation: Iron deficiency impairs hemoglobin production, limiting oxygen transport in the blood and reducing aerobic energy production. This leads to fatigue, weakness, and poor exercise performance. Adequate iron intake, especially for athletes and females, maintains optimal oxygen delivery, endurance, and recovery capacity by ensuring sufficient red blood cell function and metabolic efficiency.

Q458. Answer: B

Explanation: Water enables thermoregulation by supporting sweat evaporation, which cools the body during exercise. It prevents dangerous core temperature rises that can impair performance or cause heat-related illness. Maintaining hydration sustains cardiac output, enhances blood circulation, and ensures efficient metabolic and muscular functioning throughout prolonged physical activity in various environmental conditions.

Q459. Answer: A

Explanation: Vitamin D enhances calcium absorption by increasing intestinal transport proteins that move calcium into the bloodstream. This process maintains bone mineralization and neuromuscular function. Without adequate vitamin D, calcium uptake declines, leading to weakened bones, impaired muscle performance, and increased injury risk, especially in individuals with limited sunlight exposure or poor dietary intake.

Q460. Answer: C

Explanation: Fat provides approximately nine calories per gram, over twice the energy density of carbohydrates or proteins. This high caloric value supports long-term energy reserves and hormone regulation. While essential in moderate amounts, excessive fat consumption can hinder performance and health, emphasizing the importance of balance and quality fat sources in a training diet.

Q461. Answer: B

Explanation: The body stores carbohydrates as glycogen in the liver and skeletal muscle. During exercise, glycogen is broken down into glucose to fuel ATP production. Adequate glycogen reserves are vital for sustaining high-intensity effort and preventing fatigue, making consistent carbohydrate intake essential for energy availability and athletic endurance across all forms of training.

Q462. Answer: D

Explanation: Omega-3 fatty acids, especially EPA and DHA, support cardiovascular health by lowering triglycerides, reducing blood pressure, and decreasing inflammation. They improve endothelial function and aid in brain health and recovery. Regular consumption through fish or supplementation enhances joint mobility and overall well-being, particularly in physically active populations seeking efficient recovery and endurance support.

Q463. Answer: B

Explanation: Consuming protein soon after resistance training accelerates muscle protein synthesis, facilitating repair and growth. The body experiences heightened anabolic sensitivity post-exercise, meaning nutrient delivery efficiency peaks. Providing amino acids within this window maximizes recovery, strength development, and lean mass maintenance, supporting long-term training progression and adaptation efficiency for consistent muscular improvement.

Q464. Answer: B

Explanation: Sodium regulates extracellular fluid balance by controlling osmotic gradients across cell membranes. This ensures proper hydration, nerve transmission, and muscle function, particularly during exercise when electrolytes are lost through sweat. Maintaining sodium intake prevents hyponatremia and preserves cardiovascular stability, critical for endurance and recovery in both athletic and everyday conditions.

Q465. Answer: A

Explanation: Vitamin B12 is vital for DNA synthesis and red blood cell production, preventing anemia. It also supports myelin sheath integrity, ensuring proper nerve signal transmission. Adequate intake promotes oxygen delivery and neurological efficiency, both essential for endurance, focus, and physical performance. Deficiency commonly affects vegetarians or older adults with impaired absorption capacity.

Q466. Answer: B

Explanation: Phosphorus combines with calcium to form hydroxyapatite, the mineral compound that provides bone rigidity and strength. Balanced intake supports skeletal development and energy metabolism through ATP formation. Adequate phosphorus ensures calcium is properly utilized, promoting optimal bone density, muscle contraction, and cellular energy transfer vital for structural health and physical performance.

Q467. Answer: B

Explanation: Antioxidants such as vitamins C, E, and beta-carotene neutralize free radicals generated during metabolism and intense exercise. By reducing oxidative stress, they preserve cellular integrity, slow tissue damage, and enhance recovery. Adequate antioxidant intake supports immune resilience, endurance, and long-term health by mitigating inflammation and maintaining efficient energy production pathways during physical stress.

Q468. Answer: C

Explanation: The combination of protein and carbohydrates accelerates glycogen restoration and muscle repair after endurance events. Carbohydrates replenish energy reserves, while protein provides amino acids to rebuild tissue. Consuming this mix within the post-exercise recovery window maximizes adaptation, restores energy balance, and enhances subsequent performance capacity through synergistic nutrient utilization and hormonal response.

Q469. Answer: B

Explanation: Potassium regulates nerve impulse transmission and muscle contraction by maintaining the balance of intracellular and extracellular electrolytes. It aids in restoring normal cellular function following muscle activation. Adequate potassium intake prevents cramping, fatigue, and arrhythmias, ensuring efficient neuromuscular coordination and optimal hydration during exercise, particularly under heat or high sweat conditions.

Q470. Answer: B

Explanation: Regular, moderate water intake during exercise maintains hydration without causing gastrointestinal discomfort. This strategy sustains plasma volume, temperature control, and cardiovascular function. Continuous small sips prevent dehydration and electrolyte imbalance, improving endurance, cognitive clarity, and muscle efficiency throughout training or competition under varied environmental and intensity conditions.

Q471. Answer: B

Explanation: Glycogen acts as the body's main carbohydrate storage form, found in muscle and liver tissue. During exercise, it is broken down to glucose, supplying ATP for muscular contraction and maintaining blood glucose levels. Adequate glycogen storage enhances endurance, prevents early fatigue, and ensures sustained performance during prolonged or high-intensity activity sessions.

Q472. Answer: D

Explanation: Vitamin K is crucial for activating proteins responsible for blood clotting and bone mineralization. It supports the synthesis of prothrombin, preventing excessive bleeding, and contributes to proper calcium utilization within bone tissue. Adequate intake maintains cardiovascular and skeletal health, ensuring physiological balance and optimal recovery after training or injury situations.

Q473. Answer: B

Explanation: Sodium plays a critical role in maintaining fluid balance and nerve signaling. Excessive sweating in hot or humid conditions depletes sodium, increasing the risk of muscle cramps and dehydration. Adequate sodium intake restores electrolyte equilibrium, supports proper muscle function, and helps retain fluids, ensuring optimal thermoregulation and endurance under stressful environmental conditions.

Q474. Answer: B

Explanation: Soluble fiber binds with cholesterol in the digestive tract, reducing its absorption into the bloodstream. This mechanism lowers LDL levels and supports heart health by improving lipid profiles. Regular fiber intake from whole grains, fruits, and vegetables promotes arterial health, supports weight management, and contributes to long-term cardiovascular disease prevention.

Q475. Answer: B

Explanation: Iron forms part of hemoglobin, the oxygen-carrying component of red blood cells. It facilitates oxygen delivery to tissues, ensuring efficient aerobic energy production. Adequate iron intake supports endurance, energy levels, and recovery, while deficiency can result in fatigue and impaired performance due to decreased oxygen availability for muscular work.

Q476. Answer: A

Explanation: Omega-3 fatty acids such as EPA and DHA possess anti-inflammatory properties that aid in reducing muscle soreness and joint stiffness. They improve circulation and enhance recovery after intense exercise by minimizing oxidative stress. Regular consumption supports cardiovascular function, mental clarity, and tissue repair, improving long-term athletic performance and resilience against chronic inflammation.

Q477. Answer: B

Explanation: Phosphorus is a structural component of adenosine triphosphate (ATP), the body's main energy currency. It enables efficient energy transfer during muscular contractions and metabolic processes. Adequate phosphorus intake supports strength, recovery, and endurance by facilitating cellular respiration and maintaining acid-base balance during intense exercise and metabolic activity.

Q478. Answer: B

Explanation: Dehydration diminishes plasma volume, raising heart rate and core temperature while reducing oxygen delivery to muscles. This impairs endurance, coordination, and thermoregulation, leading to early fatigue and increased injury risk. Maintaining hydration preserves cardiovascular efficiency, electrolyte balance, and cognitive function during prolonged or high-intensity activity.

Q479. Answer: A

Explanation: Folate, or vitamin B9, is essential for DNA synthesis and cell division, particularly in tissues undergoing rapid turnover such as blood and muscle. Adequate intake ensures healthy red blood cell formation and tissue regeneration. For athletes, folate supports recovery, oxygen delivery, and overall performance by maintaining cellular growth and repair efficiency.

Q480. Answer: C

Explanation: Glucose is the exclusive and preferred energy substrate for brain function under normal conditions. The nervous system depends on a constant supply of glucose to sustain cognitive performance and neural signaling. Insufficient carbohydrate intake impairs mental clarity, coordination, and focus, making glucose critical for both exercise performance and daily physiological function.

Q481. Answer: B

Explanation: Dietary fat enables the absorption of fat-soluble vitamins (A, D, E, and K) by forming micelles within the intestines for efficient transport into the bloodstream. Without adequate fat intake, these vitamins cannot be absorbed effectively, leading to deficiencies that may impair vision, bone strength, immunity, and blood clotting processes.

Q482. Answer: B

Explanation: Proper meal timing ensures carbohydrates and proteins are available when needed for energy production, muscle repair, and recovery. Eating before training fuels performance, while post-exercise meals replenish glycogen and promote protein synthesis. Strategically scheduled meals maintain stable blood glucose levels, optimize endurance, and enhance recovery efficiency for sustained training results.

Q483. Answer: D

Explanation: Magnesium serves as a cofactor in hundreds of enzymatic reactions responsible for ATP production, muscle contraction, and nerve function. Adequate magnesium intake supports efficient energy metabolism, stabilizes heart rhythm, and promotes recovery. Deficiency can lead to fatigue, cramping, or reduced exercise capacity due to impaired metabolic and neuromuscular function.

Q484. Answer: B

Explanation: Folate plays an essential role in early fetal development by supporting DNA synthesis and cell division. Adequate folate intake before and during pregnancy prevents neural tube defects like spina bifida. This nutrient also aids red blood cell production and overall tissue health, making it vital for both maternal wellness and embryonic growth.

Q485. Answer: B

Explanation: Carbohydrates provide rapid ATP through anaerobic glycolysis during high-intensity exercise. Their fast metabolism supports explosive movements and delays fatigue when oxygen delivery is limited. Sufficient carbohydrate availability enhances performance and recovery, making glycogen stores crucial for repeated efforts and maintaining power output throughout vigorous physical activity.

Q486. Answer: A

Explanation: Vitamin C is required for collagen synthesis, forming the structural framework of connective tissue, tendons, and skin. It supports wound healing, tissue repair, and immune defense. Adequate vitamin C intake enhances recovery from training stress, prevents joint weakness, and protects against oxidative damage during intense exercise or environmental exposure.

Q487. Answer: B

Explanation: Physical training causes micro-tears in muscle fibers that require amino acids for repair and adaptation. Higher protein intake supplies these building blocks, accelerating muscle recovery, growth, and strength development. Sufficient protein consumption also preserves lean mass during caloric restriction and supports immune health in active populations.

Q488. Answer: B

Explanation: Consuming 1.0–1.5 grams of carbohydrates per kilogram of body weight within 30 minutes after training maximizes glycogen resynthesis rates. This timing takes advantage of heightened insulin sensitivity and glycogen synthase activity. Rapid replenishment restores energy reserves, enhances recovery, and prepares the body for subsequent workouts or athletic events.

Q489. Answer: C

Explanation: Protein should make up 15–25% of total daily caloric intake for active adults. This range supports muscle maintenance, recovery, and enzyme function without excessive caloric contribution. Proper protein distribution throughout meals enhances absorption, maximizes muscle protein synthesis, and contributes to satiety and metabolic balance for individuals engaging in regular physical training.

Q490. Answer: B

Explanation: Balanced macronutrient intake—adequate carbohydrates, proteins, and fats—supports energy production, tissue repair, and hormonal balance. Each macronutrient serves specific metabolic functions essential for performance and recovery. Maintaining proportional intake enhances nutrient utilization, stabilizes blood glucose, and sustains vitality across physical, cognitive, and metabolic systems for long-term wellness and optimal body function.

Q491. Answer: B

Explanation: Building rapport begins with open-ended questions and active listening, allowing the client to feel heard and respected. This approach creates trust and understanding, encouraging honest communication and long-term adherence. By prioritizing empathy and curiosity over instruction, the trainer establishes a foundation of collaboration essential for successful client-coach relationships.

Q492. Answer: D

Explanation: Paraphrasing rephrases a client's message in the coach to confirm comprehension and demonstrate attention. It strengthens mutual understanding and validates the client's feelings. This communication technique helps the client feel acknowledged, reduces misinterpretation, and reinforces the trust necessary for effective behavior change discussions and coaching outcomes.

Q493. Answer: B

Explanation: The contemplation stage occurs when clients recognize the benefits of change but have not yet committed to action, typically within six months. They weigh pros and cons of behavior modification, needing guidance, encouragement, and informational support to progress toward preparation and action. Coaches should emphasize empathy and self-efficacy to move clients forward.

Q494. Answer: B

Explanation: Motivational interviewing encourages clients to articulate their reasons for change, resolving ambivalence and enhancing intrinsic motivation. It empowers clients to make autonomous decisions by evoking their values and goals. Through empathy, reflection, and collaboration, this method strengthens commitment and fosters sustainable behavioral transformation without imposing external pressure.

Q495. Answer: C

Explanation: Open-ended questions invite thoughtful responses that encourage clients to express feelings, experiences, and motivations. This dialogue fosters deeper understanding and collaboration, giving trainers insight into client perspectives. Open-ended questioning forms the basis of motivational interviewing, supporting autonomy, engagement, and active participation in the coaching relationship.

Q496. Answer: B

Explanation: "A" in SMART stands for Attainable, emphasizing that goals must be realistic and achievable based on the client's current abilities and resources. Setting attainable goals promotes confidence and steady progress. This approach prevents frustration, enhances self-efficacy, and increases the likelihood of consistent adherence to a structured fitness plan over time.

Q497. Answer: A

Explanation: Tone of voice conveys emotion, confidence, and empathy beyond spoken words. Clients interpret tone to gauge sincerity and comfort in the coaching relationship. A calm, supportive tone establishes trust, whereas harsh or rushed speech can create tension. Managing tone effectively enhances rapport and reinforces verbal communication with warmth and authenticity.

Q498. Answer: A

Explanation: Self-efficacy improves through mastery experiences—achievable, consistent successes that reinforce a client's belief in their capabilities. Celebrating small wins enhances confidence, making larger goals seem attainable. This strategy fosters independence and persistence, key traits for sustaining long-term exercise adherence and positive behavior change beyond initial coaching supervision.

Q499. Answer: B

Explanation: When clients express frustration, trainers should acknowledge their feelings, review progress, and adjust goals if necessary. Providing empathy and encouragement renews motivation and fosters resilience. Collaborative problem-solving helps clients regain confidence in their process, reinforcing trust and commitment while maintaining alignment with realistic, measurable progress indicators.

Q500. Answer: D

Explanation: Reflective listening mirrors the client's words or emotions to demonstrate genuine understanding and empathy. It helps the client feel heard and validated, reducing defensiveness and enhancing openness to change. This technique builds rapport, deepens communication, and encourages clients to explore thoughts and behaviors more freely within a trusting relationship.

Questions (501-600)

Q501. Which statement best defines intrinsic motivation?

A. Motivation driven by external rewards
B. Desire to engage in an activity for personal satisfaction
C. Motivation stemming from fear of punishment
D. Urge to achieve recognition from others

Q502. What is the first step in the behavior change process?

A. Taking immediate action
B. Building awareness of the need for change
C. Setting performance goals
D. Creating social accountability

Q503. According to motivational interviewing, what is "rolling with resistance"?

A. Ignoring client objections
B. Arguing to enforce compliance
C. Accepting client hesitation without confrontation
D. Redirecting focus to trainer authority

Q504. What strategy enhances adherence by increasing client ownership of goals?

A. Trainer-driven programming
B. Collaborative goal setting
C. Strict accountability check-ins
D. Incentive-based motivation

Q505. What does the "O" in the OARS framework of motivational interviewing represent?

A. Observation
B. Open-ended questions
C. Outcomes
D. Organization

Q506. Which type of goal focuses on consistent effort rather than specific outcomes?

A. Process goal
B. Performance goal
C. Outcome goal
D. Extrinsic goal

Q507. How should a trainer respond when a client shares emotional barriers to exercise?

A. Shift immediately to training discussion
B. Listen empathetically and validate feelings
C. Offer medical advice
D. Downplay the client's emotions

Q508. What is the primary benefit of using positive reinforcement?

A. Increases dependence on external rewards
B. Strengthens desired behaviors through acknowledgment
C. Discourages self-reflection
D. Limits motivation to goal outcomes

Q509. What is a sign of strong trainer-client rapport?

A. Client avoids difficult discussions
B. Trainer dominates all communication
C. Client feels comfortable expressing challenges honestly
D. Client relies solely on external motivation

Q510. Which principle supports the idea that clients change behavior when they believe in their ability to succeed?
A. Self-determination
B. Self-efficacy
C. Reinforcement
D. Attribution
Q511. How should a trainer manage a client experiencing low self-esteem about fitness performance?
A. Compare them to others for motivation
B. Highlight small successes and improvements
C. Avoid addressing the issue
D. Push for immediate higher performance
Q512. Which coaching method uses empathy, collaboration, and support to guide client decisions?
A. Cognitive behavioral therapy
B. Motivational interviewing
C. Direct instruction
D. Assertive coaching
Q513. In the stages of change model, which stage involves maintaining new habits for at least six months?
A. Action
B. Termination
C. Preparation
D. Maintenance
Q514. Which component of effective communication ensures the trainer truly understands a client's message?
A. Listening to respond
B. Active listening
C. Selective hearing
D. Silence
Q515. What is the most important trainer behavior for maintaining long-term client adherence?
A. Providing consistent emotional support and encouragement
B. Continuously increasing workout difficulty
C. Monitoring only physical results
D. Focusing exclusively on nutrition plans
Q516. Which component of the OARS framework focuses on recognizing client strengths and progress?
A. Open-ended questions
B. Affirmations
C. Reflections
D. Summaries
Q517. What is the best way for a trainer to handle a client who consistently misses sessions?
A. Confront the client harshly about attendance
B. Discuss underlying barriers and adjust scheduling collaboratively
C. Apply financial penalties
D. Ignore the issue to avoid conflict
Q518. What is a primary principle of the self-determination theory?
A. External rewards are the strongest motivators
B. Autonomy, competence, and relatedness enhance motivation
C. Pressure from others improves adherence
D. Competition drives behavioral change

Q519. Which type of feedback best encourages positive behavior change?
A. Judgmental feedback
B. Vague praise
C. Constructive, specific feedback
D. Corrective-only feedback
Q520. Which of the following behaviors indicates active listening?
A. Interrupting to give advice
B. Maintaining eye contact and nodding while reflecting
C. Writing notes silently without acknowledgment
D. Waiting to speak without engagement
Q521. What is a major advantage of using the SMART goal system in coaching?
A. Encourages vague long-term visions
B. Provides structure for measurable, achievable objectives
C. Removes accountability
D. Focuses only on immediate results
Q522. When should a trainer use summaries during client communication?
A. To confirm understanding and transition topics smoothly
B. To end conversations abruptly
C. To highlight client mistakes
D. To redirect focus toward trainer expertise
Q523. Which statement best describes empathy in client communication?
A. Pity for client struggles
B. Understanding and sharing another's perspective
C. Agreement with client behavior
D. Offering solutions quickly
Q524. What is the purpose of using affirmations during motivational interviewing?
A. To manipulate client emotions
B. To build confidence and reinforce strengths
C. To correct misconceptions immediately
D. To test client knowledge
Q525. What is the most effective way to address a client's resistance to change?
A. Challenge them directly
B. Listen, validate concerns, and explore motivations collaboratively
C. Ignore objections
D. Emphasize trainer authority
Q526. What communication approach helps prevent misinterpretation of a client's message?
A. Paraphrasing
B. Giving instructions
C. Providing judgmental advice
D. Changing the subject
Q527. Which stage of change reflects a client actively modifying behavior?
A. Precontemplation
B. Contemplation
C. Action
D. Maintenance
Q528. What strategy best promotes adherence among clients new to exercise?
A. Setting overly ambitious goals
B. Focusing on early, attainable milestones

C. Comparing performance with others
D. Using only external rewards

Q529. What is the key goal of behavior modification in personal training?
A. Rapid weight loss
B. Sustainable lifestyle change
C. Maximizing exercise intensity
D. Eliminating rest periods

Q530. How should a trainer respond to client feedback about dissatisfaction with progress?
A. Reassure without analysis
B. Explore underlying reasons and adjust the program collaboratively
C. Defend the program design
D. Ignore the feedback

Q531. What is the main advantage of open-ended questioning in behavior coaching?
A. It elicits detailed client insights and encourages reflection
B. It limits client response options
C. It speeds up sessions
D. It avoids sensitive topics

Q532. What is a key trait of an effective personal trainer-client relationship?
A. Authority and control
B. Mutual respect and collaboration
C. Dependence on the trainer
D. Competitive comparison

Q533. What should a trainer emphasize to help clients develop intrinsic motivation?
A. Personal enjoyment and self-improvement
B. Competition and external rewards
C. Strict goal deadlines
D. Fear of failure

Q534. What does the "S" in SMART goals stand for?
A. Sustainable
B. Simple
C. Specific
D. Strategic

Q535. Why is empathy considered a cornerstone of effective coaching?
A. It reduces trainer accountability
B. It fosters trust and client openness
C. It encourages dependency
D. It limits emotional expression

Q536. Which of the following best demonstrates client autonomy in coaching?
A. Trainer dictates all goals
B. Client defers every decision to trainer
C. Trainer dismisses client opinions
D. Client makes informed decisions about their plan

Q537. What is a trainer's best response when a client achieves a major goal?
A. Immediately set a harder goal
B. Celebrate the success and review progress
C. Downplay the achievement to stay humble
D. Shift focus away from results

Q538. How does effective communication influence adherence?

A. Reduces trust
B. Builds understanding and motivation
C. Increases dependency
D. Limits accountability
Q539. Which coaching skill helps uncover the client's personal reasons for change?
A. Advice-giving
B. Directive feedback
C. Open-ended questioning and reflection
D. Instructional dominance
Q540. What is the most important factor in preventing client relapse?
A. Strictly increasing workout volume
B. Developing coping strategies and support systems
C. Removing all flexibility from programming
D. Avoiding progress tracking
Q541. What is the primary goal of client-centered coaching?
A. Ensure the trainer's methods are followed exactly
B. Empower clients to take ownership of their goals and decisions
C. Focus only on physical results
D. Minimize client involvement in planning
Q542. Which motivational interviewing technique helps a client explore both pros and cons of behavior change?
A. Developing discrepancy
B. Eliciting change talk
C. Affirmation
D. Goal setting
Q543. What is the most effective way to increase long-term exercise adherence?
A. Create a highly intense program
B. Build supportive relationships and realistic expectations
C. Focus solely on weight loss goals
D. Provide rigid rules without flexibility
Q544. What type of motivation is strengthened when clients identify personal values behind their goals?
A. Extrinsic motivation
B. Intrinsic motivation
C. Controlled motivation
D. Competitive motivation
Q545. When clients face setbacks, what should trainers focus on to maintain progress?
A. Blaming the client for poor discipline
B. Reframing the situation as a learning opportunity
C. Ignoring the event and moving on
D. Increasing program difficulty immediately
Q546. What is the primary benefit of setting process-oriented goals?
A. Focuses effort on daily habits and controllable actions
B. Prioritizes only final results
C. Increases dependency on external feedback
D. Reduces client accountability
Q547. Which behavior best exemplifies unconditional positive regard in coaching?
A. Criticizing clients to build resilience

B. Rewarding only when goals are met
C. Supporting clients without judgment, regardless of setbacks
D. Ignoring emotional cues

Q548. What is the best strategy for promoting behavior maintenance after goal achievement?
A. Removing accountability measures
B. Encouraging reflection and setting new challenges
C. Reducing social support
D. Returning to old habits as a "reward"

Q549. What key element should trainers use to increase client adherence during stressful periods?
A. Empathy and flexible adjustments
B. Stricter program adherence
C. Ignoring emotional factors
D. Intensifying accountability

Q550. What best describes a trainer's role in behavior change coaching?
A. Directing all decisions
B. Facilitating self-discovery and supporting autonomy
C. Imposing strict discipline
D. Providing motivational speeches only

Q551. What is the primary purpose of a fitness professional's scope of practice?
A. Define personal interests
B. Outline legal and ethical boundaries for professional actions
C. Restrict career advancement opportunities
D. Determine pay rates

Q552. When should a personal trainer refer a client to a healthcare professional?
A. When the client requests more advanced exercise options
B. When the client misses multiple sessions
C. When the client asks for nutritional supplementation advice
D. When the client shows signs of a medical condition beyond the trainer's qualifications

Q553. What is the most important reason for maintaining professional liability insurance?
A. To enhance client loyalty
B. To protect against financial loss from claims or lawsuits
C. To reduce certification renewal costs
D. To advertise professional credibility

Q554. Which document should clients sign before beginning an exercise program to acknowledge risk?
A. Par-Q only
B. Health questionnaire
C. Informed consent form
D. Liability waiver

Q555. Which organization typically provides accreditation for fitness certifications?
A. ACE
B. NCCA
C. ACSM
D. NASM

Q556. What is the primary purpose of continuing education for certified professionals?
A. Fulfill administrative requirements
B. Maintain and enhance professional knowledge and competency
C. Increase marketing exposure
D. Replace practical experience

Q557. Why should trainers maintain detailed client records?
A. To track progress, ensure accountability, and support legal protection
B. For marketing purposes
C. To share data publicly
D. To reduce client communication
Q558. What is an ethical obligation when discussing client information?
A. Share progress with peers openly
B. Keep all client information confidential unless given consent
C. Use client stories for promotion
D. Provide details to family members
Q559. What is the first step when a trainer identifies a potential conflict of interest?
A. Ignore it unless discovered by others
B. Disclose it transparently and take steps to mitigate bias
C. Continue without informing anyone
D. Delegate all related responsibilities
Q560. What is the primary benefit of professional networking in the fitness industry?
A. Competitive advantage over peers
B. Gaining social popularity
C. Expanding professional relationships and learning opportunities
D. Reducing certification requirements
Q561. Which action best demonstrates professionalism during client interactions?
A. Maintaining punctuality and preparedness for sessions
B. Allowing frequent personal interruptions
C. Using informal or casual behavior excessively
D. Sharing personal opinions frequently
Q562. What is the best way to handle a client's medical question beyond a trainer's expertise?
A. Provide advice from online sources
B. Refer them to a licensed healthcare provider
C. Offer a general answer based on experience
D. Avoid acknowledging the question
Q563. What is the ethical way to advertise personal training services?
A. Make claims based on personal opinion
B. Use truthful, evidence-based information without exaggeration
C. Promise guaranteed physical results
D. Use client transformations without consent
Q564. Which term refers to the legal responsibility to act in a reasonable and prudent manner?
A. Duty of care
B. Professional privilege
C. Client autonomy
D. Fiduciary right
Q565. What should a trainer do if a client reports new joint pain during a session?
A. Continue exercise cautiously
B. Stop activity and refer to a healthcare professional
C. Suggest over-the-counter remedies
D. Modify exercises without evaluation
Q566. What is the main purpose of a professional code of ethics?
A. Provide a marketing advantage
B. Establish standards for professional behavior and accountability

C. Replace legal regulations
D. Determine certification duration

Q567. Which factor contributes most to long-term professional success in the fitness industry?
A. Continuous learning and adaptability
B. High-intensity training programs
C. Aggressive marketing
D. Strict focus on aesthetics

Q568. What should a trainer do to ensure client confidentiality in digital communication?
A. Share progress updates on social media
B. Use secure, password-protected systems for client data
C. Store client files on public devices
D. Discuss client results in online forums

Q569. Which behavior reflects professional integrity?
A. Delivering consistent, honest communication with clients
B. Promising unrealistic results for motivation
C. Sharing competitor information
D. Ignoring feedback from supervisors

Q570. What is the purpose of informed consent in fitness assessment?
A. To gather personal opinions
B. To replace medical clearance
C. To protect only the trainer
D. To ensure clients voluntarily agree to procedures with full understanding

Q571. What is a key ethical responsibility when working with other health professionals?
A. Respect professional boundaries and collaborate appropriately
B. Compete for the same clients
C. Override medical recommendations
D. Share confidential details freely

Q572. What is the most professional way to terminate a client relationship?
A. Suddenly stop communication
B. Provide clear explanation and transition support if needed
C. Ignore missed sessions
D. Blame the client for lack of progress

Q573. Why should trainers avoid diagnosing medical conditions?
A. It's outside their scope and could result in liability
B. It builds client trust
C. It's necessary for creating programs
D. It saves clients medical costs

Q574. What is a key component of professionalism in appearance and conduct?
A. Dressing casually to seem relatable
B. Maintaining appropriate attire, hygiene, and demeanor
C. Matching clients' behavior
D. Using informal language

Q575. What is the primary reason for a trainer to pursue mentorship?
A. Gain shortcuts for career advancement
B. Receive feedback and guidance for continuous improvement
C. Replace formal education
D. Avoid personal accountability

Q576. What should a trainer do if a client requests advice on specific dietary supplements?

A. Provide personal recommendations based on experience
B. Recommend the most popular supplements online
C. Refer the client to a registered dietitian or physician
D. Sell products for commission

Q577. What is the best way for a trainer to handle a client complaint?
A. Dismiss the concern immediately
B. Listen carefully, document the issue, and address it professionally
C. Refer the client to another trainer without review
D. Ignore it to avoid confrontation

Q578. What is a trainer's ethical duty regarding client progress reporting?
A. Exaggerate results to increase motivation
B. Provide accurate, evidence-based feedback supported by data
C. Focus only on positive results
D. Withhold progress information

Q579. What is the main reason for a trainer to join a professional organization such as ACSM or NASM?
A. To receive automatic client referrals
B. To access continuing education, research, and networking
C. To replace certification exams
D. To advertise products

Q580. What is the correct action if a trainer suspects a client has an eating disorder?
A. Ignore it and continue training
B. Reduce exercise intensity temporarily
C. Offer personal nutrition tips
D. Refer the client to a qualified mental health or medical professional

Q581. Which of the following is a key principle of professional communication?
A. Speak without filtering to show honesty
B. Use clarity, empathy, and respect in all messages
C. Overwhelm clients with technical language
D. Focus communication on personal opinions

Q582. Why should trainers pursue multiple certifications or specializations?
A. To expand their knowledge and serve diverse client populations
B. To avoid continuing education
C. To increase workload without expertise
D. To appear more competitive without skill

Q583. What is the trainer's primary legal responsibility before beginning a new program with a client?
A. Collecting payment in advance
B. Obtaining informed consent and health screening documentation
C. Performing advanced medical tests
D. Designing a program immediately

Q584. What is the key reason for a trainer to maintain current CPR and AED certification?
A. To meet gym policy only
B. To be prepared to respond effectively in emergencies
C. To avoid legal paperwork
D. To market safety credentials

Q585. Which behavior demonstrates ethical practice when offering online training services?
A. Providing workouts without client screening
B. Sharing client progress publicly for marketing
C. Maintaining confidentiality and proper assessments virtually

D. Ignoring communication boundaries

Q586. What is the primary purpose of maintaining professional boundaries?

A. To limit emotional connection entirely

B. To preserve ethical integrity and prevent dual relationships

C. To make the relationship more casual

D. To avoid communication with clients

Q587. When must a trainer renew their certification to maintain active status?

A. Every two years or as specified by certifying organization

B. Every five years

C. Only upon client request

D. After leaving employment

Q588. What is the benefit of collaborating with other health professionals?

A. Enhances client outcomes through interdisciplinary expertise

B. Reduces personal responsibility

C. Eliminates the need for certification

D. Limits communication scope

Q589. What should a trainer do if a client experiences dizziness during a workout?

A. Continue at lower intensity

B. Stop exercise immediately and assess condition

C. Encourage pushing through discomfort

D. Provide water and resume activity

Q590. Which principle ensures trainers provide unbiased, fair services to all clients?

A. Equality and professionalism

B. Competitive marketing

C. Personal preference

D. Selective programming

Q591. What should a trainer do when approached about working outside their certified facility's policies?

A. Perform sessions secretly

B. Accept to gain experience

C. Ignore the policy temporarily

D. Decline and adhere to employer and legal guidelines

Q592. What is the trainer's role in helping clients interpret medical clearance forms?

A. Translate medical terminology precisely

B. Refer clients back to their healthcare provider for clarification

C. Modify clearance details

D. Disregard unclear information

Q593. What is the main purpose of obtaining a signed liability waiver?

A. Eliminate all trainer responsibility

B. Inform clients of inherent exercise risks and reduce legal exposure

C. Replace medical evaluation

D. Guarantee injury prevention

Q594. How should trainers approach cultural diversity among clients?

A. Recognize, respect, and adapt to individual differences

B. Maintain uniform methods for all clients

C. Avoid addressing cultural considerations

D. Assume all clients share the same values

Q595. Why is maintaining accurate financial records important?

A. To avoid scheduling conflicts
B. To advertise pricing online
C. To comply with tax laws and ensure transparent business practices
D. To share financial details with clients

Q596. What is the ethical trainer response when offered a financial incentive for client referrals from a supplement company?

A. Accept to increase revenue
B. Decline if it compromises impartiality or violates policy
C. Promote products without disclosure
D. Ignore potential conflict

Q597. Which professional skill enhances long-term client retention?

A. Consistent empathy and personalized support
B. Aggressive marketing and upselling
C. Rigid training routines
D. Frequent policy enforcement

Q598. What should a trainer do if they witness unethical behavior by a colleague?

A. Report the behavior through appropriate professional channels
B. Ignore it to maintain harmony
C. Join in for team unity
D. Confront publicly on social media

Q599. What is the best strategy for preventing legal issues in personal training practice?

A. Use informal agreements only
B. Avoid client assessments
C. Eliminate all communication with clients
D. Maintain documentation, insurance, and ethical standards consistently

Q600. Why should trainers participate in community fitness events or public education initiatives?

A. For personal recognition only
B. To contribute to public health and demonstrate professional leadership
C. To recruit clients aggressively
D. To avoid continuing education requirements

Answer keys and Explanations (501-600)

Q501. Answer: B
Explanation: Intrinsic motivation arises from internal enjoyment, curiosity, or fulfillment rather than external incentives. It drives long-term adherence and commitment since actions align with personal values and interests. Cultivating intrinsic motivation helps clients view exercise as rewarding in itself, making behavioral changes sustainable beyond external accountability or short-term goals.
Q502. Answer: B
Explanation: Awareness precedes all behavior change. Clients must recognize and understand why change is necessary before committing to action. This step involves education, self-reflection, and identifying barriers. Coaches can foster awareness through open dialogue and assessments, guiding clients from contemplation to preparation stages with informed motivation and personal relevance.
Q503. Answer: C
Explanation: Rolling with resistance means acknowledging and respecting client ambivalence rather than confronting it. This nonjudgmental acceptance allows clients to explore their hesitations safely, often leading to self-motivated change. By avoiding argumentation, trainers maintain rapport and empower clients to resolve internal conflicts organically through guided reflection and empathy.
Q504. Answer: B
Explanation: Collaborative goal setting involves the client actively participating in creating their objectives, fostering autonomy and commitment. When clients contribute to planning, they feel a sense of ownership and personal responsibility. This engagement builds intrinsic motivation, improves follow-through, and strengthens the overall coaching partnership for long-term adherence and satisfaction.
Q505. Answer: B
Explanation: "O" stands for Open-ended questions, which invite clients to share detailed insights about their experiences and motivations. This technique fosters reflection and exploration, providing richer context for coaching decisions. Open-ended questioning aligns with motivational interviewing principles by promoting dialogue, autonomy, and engagement, encouraging clients to identify their own reasons for change.
Q506. Answer: A
Explanation: Process goals emphasize the actions required to achieve desired outcomes, such as attending sessions or tracking meals. By focusing on daily behaviors, clients experience consistent progress and confidence. This method builds sustainable habits, reinforcing self-efficacy while reducing pressure associated with results-only benchmarks, ultimately enhancing long-term success and motivation.
Q507. Answer: B
Explanation: Empathetic listening acknowledges a client's emotions without judgment, fostering trust and openness. Validation shows respect for the client's experience, creating psychological safety for honest dialogue. This compassionate response strengthens rapport, making clients more receptive to guidance and increasing their likelihood of overcoming emotional or motivational barriers to adherence.
Q508. Answer: B
Explanation: Positive reinforcement acknowledges and rewards desired behaviors, increasing their frequency. When clients receive encouragement or recognition for progress, they associate exercise with positive emotions, enhancing commitment and consistency. This strategy supports long-term habit formation by connecting achievement to satisfaction and confidence rather than external pressure or punitive feedback.
Q509. Answer: C
Explanation: Open and honest communication signifies effective rapport. When clients feel safe to share struggles or vulnerabilities, it indicates trust and mutual respect. This transparent environment enhances

problem-solving, allowing the trainer to address barriers and adjust programs accordingly. Strong rapport fosters motivation, accountability, and long-term coaching success through authentic connection.

Q510. Answer: B

Explanation: Self-efficacy, or belief in one's ability to perform specific behaviors, predicts success in adopting and maintaining change. Enhancing this confidence through achievable challenges and consistent support encourages persistence. As clients experience mastery, their confidence grows, reinforcing motivation and adherence to exercise and lifestyle modifications over the long term.

Q511. Answer: B

Explanation: Recognizing and celebrating small victories fosters a sense of competence and progress, building confidence and motivation. Positive reinforcement shifts focus from shortcomings to achievement, helping clients develop a healthier self-image. This supportive approach strengthens emotional resilience and promotes consistent engagement, crucial for sustainable behavior change and self-belief development.

Q512. Answer: B

Explanation: Motivational interviewing employs empathy, open dialogue, and autonomy-supportive communication to help clients explore motivations and overcome ambivalence. It strengthens self-determination by aligning goals with personal values. This collaborative style builds trust and empowerment, promoting sustained commitment to lifestyle change through intrinsic motivation rather than external enforcement or authority-driven direction.

Q513. Answer: D

Explanation: The maintenance stage begins after six months of consistent behavior change. Clients focus on reinforcing habits and preventing relapse. Ongoing support, goal refinement, and reinforcement help sustain motivation. Trainers assist by providing accountability, celebrating continued progress, and ensuring that the new lifestyle becomes permanent and self-sustaining over time.

Q514. Answer: B

Explanation: Active listening involves full engagement, concentration, and feedback, ensuring the trainer accurately comprehends the client's words and emotions. This attentive approach fosters empathy, builds trust, and prevents misunderstandings. By summarizing or reflecting responses, the trainer validates the client's perspective and strengthens communication effectiveness within the coaching relationship.

Q515. Answer: A

Explanation: Consistent encouragement and emotional support nurture motivation, accountability, and connection. Clients who feel valued and supported are more likely to remain engaged and persistent through challenges. This empathetic approach fosters resilience, reinforces intrinsic motivation, and transforms exercise adherence into a sustainable lifestyle rather than a short-term commitment.

Q516. Answer: B

Explanation: Affirmations acknowledge client efforts, strengths, and accomplishments, reinforcing self-efficacy and confidence. This positive reinforcement encourages continued effort and highlights progress, making clients feel competent and valued. By focusing on what the client does well, affirmations enhance motivation, solidify rapport, and create an empowering atmosphere that supports ongoing behavior change.

Q517. Answer: B

Explanation: Addressing attendance issues through empathetic discussion allows the trainer to identify underlying barriers such as time constraints or motivation. Collaborative problem-solving respects the client's circumstances while maintaining accountability. Adjusting scheduling or strategies demonstrates flexibility and care, increasing adherence by aligning the program with realistic lifestyle conditions.

Q518. Answer: B

Explanation: Self-determination theory emphasizes three key psychological needs—autonomy, competence, and relatedness—as foundations for intrinsic motivation. When clients feel empowered, capable, and supported, they are more likely to sustain healthy behaviors voluntarily. Fostering these elements creates internal drive, resulting in stronger adherence and satisfaction with long-term behavior change outcomes.

Q519. Answer: C

Explanation: Constructive feedback focuses on specific, actionable details while reinforcing effort and improvement. This approach supports learning and growth rather than criticism, helping clients identify strengths and development areas clearly. Balanced feedback enhances confidence, builds trust, and encourages continuous engagement in behavior change processes through positive reinforcement and guidance.

Q520. Answer: B

Explanation: Active listening involves attentive body language, verbal affirmations, and reflective responses. Maintaining eye contact and nodding demonstrates presence and empathy, encouraging open dialogue. This behavior assures clients they are heard and valued, strengthening trust and communication effectiveness in the coaching relationship and improving long-term adherence to goals.

Q521. Answer: B

Explanation: The SMART framework ensures goals are Specific, Measurable, Attainable, Relevant, and Time-bound, offering clear direction and progress tracking. This structure fosters accountability, confidence, and consistency. It allows both client and trainer to measure achievement objectively, making adjustments as needed to sustain motivation and optimize success in behavior modification programs.

Q522. Answer: A

Explanation: Summaries consolidate discussions, confirming comprehension and highlighting key themes or commitments. This communication tool ensures both trainer and client share mutual understanding, helping guide transitions between topics effectively. Summarizing reinforces active listening, validates client input, and strengthens collaboration, keeping sessions organized and client-centered throughout the coaching process.

Q523. Answer: B

Explanation: Empathy involves perceiving and understanding the client's experiences and emotions from their point of view. It creates a foundation of trust, demonstrating care without judgment. This relational connection enhances openness and emotional safety, allowing clients to communicate authentically and engage more deeply in the behavior change process.

Q524. Answer: B

Explanation: Affirmations highlight client progress, positive behaviors, and inner resources, reinforcing confidence and belief in their ability to succeed. This approach nurtures self-efficacy and intrinsic motivation. By recognizing genuine effort and capability, affirmations enhance trust, empower clients, and sustain engagement in continuous behavioral improvement and habit formation.

Q525. Answer: B

Explanation: Responding to resistance with empathy and curiosity helps clients feel understood and supported. Exploring their motivations collaboratively identifies underlying barriers without confrontation. This approach transforms resistance into opportunity for reflection, empowering clients to develop personal reasons for change and increasing readiness to act voluntarily.

Q526. Answer: A

Explanation: Paraphrasing involves restating a client's message in the trainer's own words to ensure clarity and mutual understanding. It prevents miscommunication, demonstrates attentiveness, and confirms accurate interpretation of key points. This skill validates client perspectives and strengthens the connection between coach and client through active, reflective communication.

Q527. Answer: C

Explanation: The action stage occurs when clients are actively engaging in new behaviors, typically within the past six months. They implement strategies, build consistency, and receive reinforcement to prevent relapse. Trainers support this stage through encouragement, monitoring progress, and reinforcing new habits to transition effectively into long-term maintenance.

Q528. Answer: B

Explanation: Early, attainable milestones create positive reinforcement and visible success, boosting self-efficacy. Small wins generate motivation and confidence, encouraging persistence through initial challenges. Trainers who emphasize incremental progress help clients internalize success, laying the foundation for consistent behavior and long-term exercise adherence.

Q529. Answer: B

Explanation: Behavior modification focuses on developing consistent, sustainable lifestyle habits that promote long-term health rather than short-term results. It involves gradual adjustments in mindset and routines. The goal is lasting adherence, empowering clients to maintain positive behaviors autonomously and reducing dependence on external motivation or supervision.

Q530. Answer: B

Explanation: Acknowledging dissatisfaction and discussing possible causes openly demonstrates respect and adaptability. Collaborative problem-solving engages the client in refining their plan, increasing ownership and motivation. This transparent approach builds trust, ensures alignment with goals, and strengthens commitment to improvement through mutual understanding and action adjustments.

Q531. Answer: A

Explanation: Open-ended questions encourage clients to think deeply and express personal motivations, barriers, and goals. This dialogue reveals valuable psychological and emotional context, enabling tailored interventions. Such questions foster autonomy and engagement, empowering clients to explore their behavior patterns and drive meaningful, self-directed change under supportive guidance.

Q532. Answer: B

Explanation: A successful trainer-client relationship is built on mutual respect, collaboration, and open communication. These qualities create trust, allowing the client to feel supported and valued. Cooperative relationships encourage accountability and empowerment, helping clients take ownership of their fitness journey and achieve sustainable progress with shared responsibility.

Q533. Answer: A

Explanation: Intrinsic motivation thrives when clients connect exercise to personal satisfaction, enjoyment, and self-growth. Trainers can highlight how fitness enhances daily life, mood, and confidence, fostering internal reward. This mindset supports lasting adherence and self-driven progress, as motivation stems from internal values rather than temporary external incentives.

Q534. Answer: C

Explanation: “S” stands for Specific, ensuring goals are clearly defined and measurable. Specificity clarifies expectations, enabling focused effort and accountability. Clearly articulated goals provide direction and motivation, reducing ambiguity and supporting precise tracking of progress, which enhances adherence and confidence in achieving desired outcomes.

Q535. Answer: B

Explanation: Empathy builds trust by showing genuine understanding and concern for a client’s experiences. When clients feel heard without judgment, they become more receptive to guidance. This emotional connection strengthens rapport, promotes honesty, and fosters an environment where meaningful, sustainable behavior change can flourish through collaborative problem-solving.

Q536. Answer: D

Explanation: Autonomy empowers clients to take active roles in their fitness journey, making decisions that align with their values and readiness. Trainers facilitate choice and education, fostering independence and self-confidence. When clients experience control over their process, adherence and satisfaction increase through internal motivation and responsibility.

Q537. Answer: B

Explanation: Celebrating accomplishments reinforces positive behavior and validates effort, boosting self-efficacy. Reviewing progress acknowledges growth and clarifies next steps, maintaining momentum toward new goals. Recognition strengthens motivation, builds confidence, and fosters long-term engagement by linking achievement to personal value and satisfaction rather than external validation alone.

Q538. Answer: B

Explanation: Clear, empathetic communication strengthens trust and ensures mutual understanding between trainer and client. This dynamic boosts motivation, engagement, and accountability by aligning goals with client needs. Effective communication allows adjustments and feedback to be delivered constructively, enhancing adherence and satisfaction with the fitness experience.

Q539. Answer: C

Explanation: Open-ended questions and reflective listening encourage clients to articulate their personal motivations and values. These insights reveal the internal drivers behind behavior change, guiding the trainer in tailoring strategies that align with what truly matters to the client, thus enhancing intrinsic motivation and commitment.

Q540. Answer: B

Explanation: Relapse prevention relies on preparing clients to handle setbacks through coping mechanisms and social support. Identifying potential barriers and developing realistic responses builds resilience. Supportive networks and proactive planning enable clients to maintain progress even when motivation wanes, ensuring long-term behavioral consistency and adherence.

Q541. Answer: B

Explanation: Client-centered coaching prioritizes autonomy by empowering clients to make informed decisions aligned with their values and goals. This approach enhances motivation, accountability, and confidence. When clients feel ownership of their progress, they are more committed and consistent, resulting in sustainable behavior change and stronger long-term adherence to fitness and lifestyle programs.

Q542. Answer: A

Explanation: Developing discrepancy encourages clients to examine the gap between their current behaviors and desired outcomes. This reflective process heightens self-awareness, allowing clients to recognize inconsistencies and internalize their reasons for change. By guiding clients to discover personal motivation through reflection, trainers promote meaningful and self-driven commitment to action.

Q543. Answer: B

Explanation: Long-term adherence depends on supportive coaching relationships that foster trust, motivation, and realistic goal-setting. When clients experience encouragement and achievable progress, they remain engaged and confident. Building strong rapport, celebrating milestones, and adapting programs to individual needs ensures consistency and sustained participation in exercise behavior over time.

Q544. Answer: B

Explanation: Intrinsic motivation arises when clients connect exercise to deeply held personal values and enjoyment rather than external rewards. Recognizing how physical activity supports self-fulfillment fosters genuine engagement. This internal drive sustains adherence, as clients pursue goals for satisfaction, self-improvement, and overall well-being rather than outside validation or pressure.

Q545. Answer: B

Explanation: Reframing setbacks as opportunities for learning and growth transforms negative experiences into motivation. This perspective builds resilience, self-efficacy, and problem-solving skills. Trainers who normalize challenges help clients maintain confidence and commitment, reinforcing adaptive thinking that sustains behavioral consistency even when progress temporarily slows.

Q546. Answer: A

Explanation: Process-oriented goals emphasize consistent, controllable behaviors—like attending workouts or logging nutrition—that build lasting habits. This focus helps clients celebrate small, actionable steps, reinforcing self-efficacy and motivation. By shifting attention from distant outcomes to immediate progress, process goals create sustainable behavioral momentum essential for long-term success.

Q547. Answer: C

Explanation: Unconditional positive regard means accepting and supporting clients without judgment, even when they struggle. This compassionate stance creates psychological safety and fosters trust. Clients who feel valued despite setbacks are more open to feedback and more likely to stay engaged in the coaching process, facilitating deeper commitment to change.

Q548. Answer: B

Explanation: Reflecting on accomplishments reinforces self-efficacy, while setting new, progressive goals maintains motivation and focus. Continuous challenges prevent complacency and solidify long-term behavioral consistency. This forward-focused approach ensures clients remain engaged, viewing health and fitness as an evolving journey rather than a temporary task.

Q549. Answer: A

Explanation: Demonstrating empathy and adapting the program to accommodate stress enhances client resilience and adherence. Flexibility shows understanding, reducing perceived pressure while maintaining momentum. This supportive adjustment helps clients stay consistent through challenges, preserving motivation and commitment by aligning fitness with realistic life circumstances and emotional readiness.

Q550. Answer: B

Explanation: The trainer's role in behavior change is to guide clients toward self-awareness, helping them identify their motivations and solutions. By facilitating autonomy and supporting personal discovery, trainers empower clients to take control of their goals. This collaborative approach enhances intrinsic motivation, long-term adherence, and sustainable lifestyle transformation rooted in self-efficacy.

Q551. Answer: B

Explanation: The scope of practice defines the legal and ethical parameters within which fitness professionals must operate. It ensures client safety, maintains professional credibility, and prevents liability by restricting trainers to activities aligned with their education and credentials. Adhering to scope of practice upholds industry standards and promotes trust among clients and allied health professionals.

Q552. Answer: D

Explanation: Trainers must refer clients to licensed healthcare providers if symptoms, pain, or conditions arise outside their expertise. This ensures ethical practice and client safety. Referrals demonstrate professional responsibility and protect both the client and trainer from inappropriate or unsafe interventions that exceed the trainer's scope of knowledge or certification.

Q553. Answer: B

Explanation: Liability insurance shields trainers from financial risk if a client files a claim related to injury, negligence, or breach of contract. It covers legal fees and settlements, ensuring protection and peace of mind. Maintaining current insurance is a best practice and often required by employers or training facilities for professional operation.

Q554. Answer: C

Explanation: Informed consent educates clients about potential risks, benefits, and expectations of exercise participation. Signing this form ensures that clients understand the program's demands and accept responsibility for voluntary participation. It protects both the client and trainer legally while promoting transparency and ethical practice standards within the professional relationship.

Q555. Answer: B

Explanation: The National Commission for Certifying Agencies (NCCA) accredits fitness and health-related certifications to ensure they meet rigorous industry standards for competency and validity. Accreditation confirms that the certification reflects evidence-based practices and professional accountability, reinforcing the credibility and recognition of certified personal trainers in the fitness industry.

Q556. Answer: B

Explanation: Continuing education ensures that fitness professionals remain up-to-date with evolving research, technologies, and best practices. It reinforces ethical responsibility to provide safe, effective, and evidence-based training. Ongoing learning enhances expertise, fosters professional growth, and preserves certification status through compliance with renewal requirements mandated by accrediting bodies.

Q557. Answer: A

Explanation: Accurate recordkeeping documents assessments, progress, and communications, serving as both a professional tool and legal safeguard. It enables program adjustments, ensures continuity, and protects against liability disputes. Maintaining organized, confidential records reflects professionalism, supports evidence-based decision-making, and upholds ethical standards in client management.

Q558. Answer: B

Explanation: Client confidentiality is a core ethical principle requiring trainers to protect personal information unless explicit written consent is provided. Maintaining privacy builds trust and complies with professional and legal standards. Unauthorized disclosure violates ethical codes and may result in disciplinary or legal consequences for the trainer.

Q559. Answer: B

Explanation: Transparency ensures ethical integrity when conflicts of interest arise. By disclosing potential biases—financial, personal, or professional—a trainer maintains client trust and avoids unethical influence. Managing or removing the conflict preserves impartiality and aligns with professional codes of conduct promoting fairness and honesty in all client interactions.

Q560. Answer: C

Explanation: Professional networking connects trainers with peers, mentors, and experts across related fields, facilitating knowledge exchange and collaboration. These relationships open opportunities for continuing education, referrals, and career advancement. Networking fosters community engagement and helps trainers remain informed about industry trends and best practices, enhancing professional development.

Q561. Answer: A

Explanation: Punctuality and preparedness show respect for clients' time and commitment, reinforcing professionalism. Consistent organization, attention to detail, and reliability enhance credibility and trust. These behaviors reflect dedication to client outcomes, creating a positive experience and strong professional reputation in the fitness environment.

Q562. Answer: B

Explanation: Trainers must remain within their defined scope of practice and refer clients to appropriate medical professionals for conditions or inquiries beyond their qualifications. This ensures ethical compliance and client safety. By collaborating with healthcare providers, trainers demonstrate responsibility and maintain professional credibility through adherence to evidence-based practices.

Q563. Answer: B

Explanation: Ethical marketing requires accuracy and honesty in all promotional materials. Trainers must avoid exaggerated claims, misleading guarantees, or unauthorized testimonials. Providing factual, evidence-based information establishes credibility and aligns with professional standards. Ethical advertising builds long-term trust and supports the integrity of the fitness industry.

Q564. Answer: A

Explanation: Duty of care obligates trainers to uphold professional standards and protect clients from foreseeable harm by acting responsibly and competently. It ensures that trainers prioritize safety, use appropriate judgment, and maintain current knowledge. Fulfilling this duty reinforces trust, professionalism, and ethical accountability in every training relationship.

Q565. Answer: B

Explanation: When new pain arises, the safest action is to stop the exercise immediately and refer the client to a healthcare provider. Trainers should never diagnose or treat pain. Prompt referral ensures client safety, prevents exacerbation, and demonstrates professional responsibility consistent with the trainer's scope of practice.

Q566. Answer: B

Explanation: A professional code of ethics sets behavioral expectations, guiding trainers in decision-making and client interactions. It defines integrity, respect, confidentiality, and competence, promoting ethical consistency. Adherence to this code strengthens public confidence, ensures fair treatment, and maintains the professional credibility of certified personal trainers.

Q567. Answer: A

Explanation: Continuous education and adaptability allow professionals to stay aligned with current research and client needs. The evolving nature of fitness science demands flexibility and commitment to learning. Trainers who refine their skills remain competitive, capable, and effective, ensuring sustained success and client satisfaction over time.

Q568. Answer: B

Explanation: Using secure, password-protected software and encrypted communication preserves client privacy and complies with data protection laws. This safeguards sensitive information from unauthorized access. Maintaining digital confidentiality demonstrates professionalism, reinforces client trust, and fulfills ethical and legal obligations in managing electronic records responsibly.

Q569. Answer: A

Explanation: Integrity involves honesty, transparency, and consistency in professional conduct. Trainers who communicate truthfully and maintain ethical standards foster credibility and long-term client relationships. Integrity builds reputation and trust, ensuring alignment between professional actions and moral responsibility within all aspects of practice.

Q570. Answer: D

Explanation: Informed consent ensures clients understand the nature, risks, and benefits of assessment procedures and agree to participate voluntarily. This process promotes transparency and autonomy, protecting both client and trainer legally and ethically. It confirms that participation is based on full awareness and informed decision-making.

Q571. Answer: A

Explanation: Ethical collaboration involves respecting each professional's scope of practice while cooperating for client benefit. Trainers should communicate openly, exchange relevant information responsibly, and uphold confidentiality. Maintaining clear professional boundaries fosters mutual respect, improves client outcomes, and strengthens multidisciplinary teamwork.

Q572. Answer: B

Explanation: Ending a client relationship ethically involves transparent communication, clear reasoning, and, if appropriate, referral or transition guidance. This approach ensures professionalism and preserves goodwill. Maintaining respect during termination protects reputation, avoids misunderstandings, and upholds ethical accountability within the client-trainer relationship.

Q573. Answer: A

Explanation: Diagnosing medical conditions exceeds a trainer's legal scope and may result in serious liability or harm. Trainers should instead recognize warning signs and refer clients to qualified healthcare professionals. This ethical practice prioritizes client safety and maintains professional integrity, ensuring collaboration within appropriate expertise boundaries.

Q574. Answer: B

Explanation: Professional appearance and demeanor communicate competence, respect, and reliability. Proper attire and hygiene create a positive impression and foster confidence in clients. Consistently maintaining professional standards of presentation reflects commitment to excellence and enhances the trainer's credibility within fitness environments.

Q575. Answer: B

Explanation: Mentorship provides valuable insights, constructive feedback, and professional guidance from experienced peers. It enhances learning beyond formal education, helping trainers refine skills, build confidence, and navigate career challenges effectively. Engaging with mentors fosters growth, ethical awareness, and long-term professional success through shared expertise and support.

Q576. Answer: C

Explanation: Trainers must remain within their scope of practice and refer supplement inquiries to registered dietitians or physicians. This ensures evidence-based recommendations and client safety while avoiding liability. Collaboration with qualified nutrition professionals demonstrates ethical integrity and supports comprehensive care through interdisciplinary cooperation.

Q577. Answer: B

Explanation: Addressing complaints promptly and respectfully demonstrates professionalism and commitment to service quality. Listening attentively and documenting details ensures transparency and accountability. By responding with empathy and solutions, trainers maintain trust, improve client satisfaction, and strengthen their professional reputation through responsible conflict resolution.

Q578. Answer: B

Explanation: Trainers are ethically obligated to report progress truthfully using valid assessments and objective data. Accurate feedback reinforces trust and helps guide programming decisions. Transparency supports client understanding of progress and areas for improvement, promoting accountability, informed decision-making, and professional credibility in all communications.

Q579. Answer: B

Explanation: Membership in professional organizations offers access to ongoing education, industry research, and networking opportunities. These resources keep trainers current on best practices, scientific advancements, and ethical standards. Engaging with professional communities enhances credibility, collaboration, and continuous learning throughout a fitness career.

Q580. Answer: D

Explanation: Trainers must refer clients exhibiting signs of eating disorders to licensed mental health or medical professionals. Early referral ensures appropriate diagnosis and treatment while maintaining professional boundaries. Recognizing signs compassionately and facilitating support demonstrates ethical responsibility and prioritizes client well-being above training goals.

Q581. Answer: B

Explanation: Professional communication combines clarity, empathy, and respect to ensure understanding and maintain a positive client relationship. Trainers who communicate effectively foster trust, motivation, and cooperation. This balanced approach demonstrates professionalism, enhances instruction comprehension, and prevents misunderstandings in both verbal and written interactions.

Q582. Answer: A

Explanation: Earning specialized credentials broadens expertise, allowing trainers to serve diverse populations such as older adults, athletes, or those with medical considerations. Continuous skill development enhances service quality and career opportunities. Specialization demonstrates commitment to professional growth and reinforces credibility across specialized domains of health and fitness.

Q583. Answer: B

Explanation: Trainers must complete informed consent and pre-participation health screenings before initiating exercise programs. These documents verify readiness, identify potential risks, and establish legal protection for both parties. This process ensures safety, informed participation, and ethical compliance with professional standards and regulatory expectations.

Q584. Answer: B

Explanation: CPR and AED certifications equip trainers to act quickly and appropriately in life-threatening situations. Being prepared ensures client safety and fulfills professional responsibility. Maintaining these credentials demonstrates readiness, adherence to industry standards, and commitment to public health and emergency preparedness during sessions.

Q585. Answer: C

Explanation: Ethical online coaching mirrors in-person professionalism—protecting privacy, performing health screenings, and respecting communication boundaries. Trainers must ensure digital platforms are secure and maintain professional conduct throughout virtual interactions. Upholding confidentiality and client safety reinforces credibility and builds trust in digital service delivery.

Q586. Answer: B

Explanation: Professional boundaries distinguish the coach-client relationship from personal interactions, ensuring impartiality and ethical conduct. Maintaining boundaries prevents conflicts of interest or inappropriate dual relationships. This structure fosters trust, professionalism, and respect, supporting effective coaching dynamics and protecting both client and trainer integrity.

Q587. Answer: A

Explanation: Most accrediting organizations, including NASM and ACSM, require certification renewal every two years to ensure professionals remain current with evolving research and best practices. Regular renewal demonstrates accountability, continuous learning, and adherence to established professional competency standards critical for maintaining credibility.

Q588. Answer: A

Explanation: Collaboration among trainers, dietitians, and healthcare professionals integrates diverse expertise to optimize client care. It ensures comprehensive support across fitness, nutrition, and medical domains. This teamwork promotes safety, consistency, and enhanced results while strengthening credibility through evidence-based, cooperative professional relationships.

Q589. Answer: B

Explanation: Dizziness is a potential sign of overexertion or medical distress. The trainer must stop the session immediately, assess symptoms, and, if necessary, refer for medical evaluation. Acting promptly ensures client safety and aligns with ethical duty of care and emergency response procedures.

Q590. Answer: A

Explanation: Upholding equality and professionalism guarantees that all clients receive fair treatment regardless of age, gender, background, or ability. This inclusive approach reinforces ethical responsibility, promotes diversity, and reflects respect for all individuals. Equal service delivery strengthens public trust and enhances the reputation of the profession.

Q591. Answer: D

Explanation: Trainers must respect facility policies and legal contracts that govern employment. Acting outside official procedures can result in disciplinary action or liability. Adherence to policy ensures compliance, maintains integrity, and preserves professional standing within the organization and the broader fitness community.

Q592. Answer: B

Explanation: Trainers should not interpret or alter medical recommendations but refer clients to their healthcare provider for clarification. This ensures proper communication between medical and fitness professionals, maintaining safety and alignment with the client's health status. Respecting expertise boundaries upholds ethical and legal responsibilities.

Q593. Answer: B

Explanation: A liability waiver educates clients on potential exercise risks and helps protect trainers from certain legal claims. While it doesn't eliminate responsibility, it reinforces transparency and informed participation. This document promotes accountability, ensures ethical standards, and safeguards both client and professional during training activities.

Q594. Answer: A

Explanation: Respecting cultural diversity means acknowledging unique values, communication styles, and preferences. Trainers who adapt appropriately foster inclusivity and trust, ensuring equitable service. This cultural competence enhances rapport, supports client comfort, and aligns with professional ethics promoting fairness and personalized care.

Q595. Answer: C

Explanation: Accurate financial records document income, expenses, and transactions, ensuring compliance with tax and business regulations. Proper accounting promotes transparency, prevents disputes, and protects against legal or financial complications. Maintaining organized records reflects professionalism and responsible management in operating a fitness business.

Q596. Answer: B

Explanation: Accepting incentives may present conflicts of interest or bias client recommendations. Ethical trainers decline such offers unless transparency and compliance with policy are ensured. Prioritizing client welfare over personal gain maintains integrity and aligns with professional codes emphasizing honesty and impartiality.

Q597. Answer: A

Explanation: Empathy and personalized attention strengthen emotional connection and trust between trainer and client. Recognizing individual goals and challenges enhances satisfaction and loyalty. This client-centered approach fosters open communication, motivation, and sustained relationships that drive long-term retention and referral growth.

Q598. Answer: A

Explanation: Reporting unethical conduct through proper internal or professional channels preserves integrity and accountability. Trainers have an ethical duty to protect clients and uphold industry standards. Confidential reporting prevents harm, ensures fairness, and demonstrates responsibility to the profession and the public.

Q599. Answer: D

Explanation: Consistent documentation, liability insurance, and adherence to ethical guidelines minimize legal risks. These practices provide a verifiable record of professional conduct, support informed consent, and reinforce trust. Preventive legal diligence protects both clients and professionals from disputes or claims of negligence.

Q600. Answer: B

Explanation: Involvement in community health initiatives demonstrates leadership, commitment, and social responsibility. Trainers who engage in outreach promote fitness awareness, inspire healthier lifestyles, and elevate the profession's public image. Contributing expertise to community wellness aligns with ethical service and enhances professional reputation.

Made in United States
Orlando, FL
04 November 2026

90201063R00090